FIXING YOU®

BOOKS IN THE **FIXING YOU** SERIES:

Back Pain

Neck Pain & Headaches

Shoulder & Elbow Pain

Hip & Knee Pain

Foot & Ankle Pain

Back Pain During Pregnancy

FIXING YOU®:
HIP &
KNEE PAIN

SELF-TREATMENT FOR
HIP PAIN, BURSITIS,
ANTERIOR KNEE PAIN,
HAMSTRING STRAINS,
AND OTHER DIAGNOSES

RICK OLDERMAN
MSPT, CPT

BOONE
PUBLISHING, LLC

2011 Boone Publishing, LLC

Boone Publishing, LLC

Editor: Lauren Manoy (lauren.manoy@gmail.com)
Interior Layout & Design: Lauren Manoy (lauren.manoy@gmail.com)
Medical Illustrations: Martin Huber (mdhuber@gmail.com)
Exercise Photographs: MaryLynn Gillaspie Photography

Boone Publishing, LLC
www.BoonePublishing.com

Library of Congress Control Number: 2009922376

Library of Congress Subject Heading:
1. Hip Pain—Physical Therapy—Treatment—Handbooks, manuals, etc. 2.
Knee Pain—Physical Therapy—Treatment—Handbooks, manuals, etc. 3.
Hip Pain—Popular Works. 4. Knee Pain—Popular Works 5. Hip—Care &
Hygiene—Popular Works. 6. Knee—Care & Hygiene—Popular Works. 7.
Hip Pain—Exercise Therapy. 8. Knee Pain—Exercise Therapy. 9. Self-care,
Health—Handbooks, manuals, etc. 10. Hip Pain—Alternative Treatment. 11.
Knee Pain—Alternative Treatment. 12. Hip Pain—Exercise Therapy. 13. Knee
Pain—Exercise Therapy. 14. Hip Pain—Prevention. 15. Knee Pain—Preven-
tion. I. Title: Fixing you: hip & knee pain. II. Olderman, Rick. III. Title.

ISBN 978-0-9821937-2-3

Printed in the United States of America

Version 1.0

ACKNOWLEDGEMENTS

In science and medicine, we build on the shoulders of those who have discovered truths before us. Writing the Fixing You series has been no different. I would like to deeply thank Dr. Shirley A. Sahrmann for her breakthrough text, *Diagnosis and Treatment of Movement Impairment Syndromes*, on which the subject of this series is based. Were it not for her textbook and seminars, which I have immensely enjoyed, I would not have been able to write the Fixing You series, much less help so many people with chronic pain or injuries. Dr. Sahrmann is a rare breed of lecturer, therapist, and researcher with a sharp mind and wit to match. Her depth of knowledge in all things musculoskeletal and biomechanical leaves me speechless.

Additionally, I would like to thank Florence Kendall, Elizabeth McCreary, and Patricia Provance for their classic text, *Muscles: Testing and Function, with Posture and Pain*. This book has been a tectonic plate on which our understanding of orthopedic physical therapy stands.

THANK YOU!

I would like to thank Lauren Manoy for painstakingly editing this book. She has meticulously sifted through this information and helped me strike a balance between delivering technical information and making it digestible for you, my reader.

Thank you to Michelle for being my rehabilitation model as well as a star client!

Thank you Ken Margel and Scott Sturgis for shooting the rehabilitation video for me.

Thank you MaryLynn for the wonderful photos.

Thank you to Martin Huber for the illuminating medical illustrations.

Thank you to all my patients and clients who unwittingly served as my guinea pigs and those who wittingly modeled for pictures!

Last, thank you to my family for putting up with long hours of writing, meetings, and physical therapy speak.

This is dedicated to David.

CONTENTS

INTRODUCTION

Thirty spokes converge upon a single hub,
it is on the hole in the center that the use
of the cart hinges.

We make a vessel from a lump of clay,
it is the empty space within that vessel
that makes it useful.

We make doors and windows for a room,
but it is these empty spaces that make
the room livable.

Thus, while the tangible has advantages,
it is the intangible that makes it useful.

—**LAO TZU**

Fixing injuries requires, among other things, an understanding of anatomy and biomechanics. That is why this book and the others in my Fixing You series presents the Fixing You approach using clear and easy-to-follow language, case studies from my practice, and pictures and diagrams to guide you, the reader, in fixing your pain. My goal is to help you visualize exactly how your body works and what is going wrong when you experience pain. When you understand and can see clearly what causes your pain, you can develop and implement a plan to fix it using the exercises and tips outlined in the Fixing You series. But knowledge is only half the answer to the problem of chronic pain. True healing also requires adjusting your mental processes to work for you, not against you.

Attention to your body and how it is or isn't working is absolutely necessary to recover from chronic pain. In fact, lack of attention is a common factor in most peoples' health issues. Developing body awareness is often the most difficult—and most important—aspect of healing from chronic pain.

Intention is another intangible but crucial aspect of healing. Harnessing your intention—your singular focus toward getting better—will reap enormous dividends. Visualize it, verbalize it, write it down, and live as if you are getting better every day; in the process you will discover which habits are counter to your goals. Once you identify these habits, you can change them. Each change will reinforce your intention. The Fixing You series presents you with knowledge about the anatomy and biomechanics of injuries, and your attention and intention makes that information useful.

A NEW PERSPECTIVE

Since graduating from physical therapy school in 1996, I've spent hundreds of hours in continuing education classes and read countless professional journal articles and books that all attempted to answer these questions: Why do we have pain, and how do we fix it? I quickly realized there was more to injuries and healing than what I was taught in the courses I had been taking, although each had a piece of the puzzle. I realized that I needed a more complete understanding not only of how muscles and bones worked, but how they worked together to create movement.

Throughout my early years as a physical therapist, I tried one person's approach here and another's technique there. These various ideas about how to treat pain sometimes worked temporarily, but usually my clients didn't present or respond exactly like the case studies in the courses. Wanting to help people and not having the answers was frustrating. So I resolved to observe my patients closely, and I started to see the following patterns emerge:

- Patients resolving back pain using methods counter to traditional approaches.

- Chronic hamstring tightness and strains in athletes with strong hamstrings.

- Correcting structural issues in people with chronic neck pain and headaches only to have them return again and again.

- Knee pain in people whose leg muscles were strong and had good range of motion.

- Repeated straining of shoulder muscles in athletes whose musculature was strong.

In the meantime, I began exploring personal training over several years while working at an exclusive fitness club in Denver, Colorado. I had exercised all my life and found my work as a physical therapist limiting in terms of my career or life goals. Personal training seemed to be a natural extension of my interests in working with people within a larger spectrum than just treating them in a clinic.

My first client was a woman who was unable to raise her arm over her head. I reviewed her workout and found that she was doing all the wrong exercises for someone with her issues.

"Doesn't this workout hurt you?" I asked her.

"Of course it does," she replied. "Isn't it supposed to be painful?"

"No, it should be pain free," I said.

"What about 'no pain, no gain'?" she asked.

"No pain, no gain" is much like Nike's slogan "Just Do It"—you must understand that you still have to check yourself to be sure what you are doing is not harmful.

What may help one client may hurt another. I knew then that the fitness field needed more physical therapists. We are trained to not only assess joint and muscle function but to extrapolate that information into a performance model for sport, work, or just plain healthy living. Currently, the fitness industry includes personal trainers and Pilates, aerobic, and Yoga instructors who are trying to help clients in pain but who have limited knowledge of anatomy or the optimal biomechanics of a healthy body—much less an injured one.

Working as a personal trainer gave me access to a type of injury that I hadn't much experience with—chronic pain. As a physical therapist in a sports and orthopedic clinic, the majority of my patients had acute injuries or surgical repairs. But there are thousands of people—if not millions—in the clubs and corporations across the United States who are exercising or working in pain, fighting chronic injuries that they've been dealing with for years, and trying to make themselves better. I know because I quickly became the busiest and highest-producing trainer/therapist at the club during my tenure there. At the time, and even now to a large extent, most people do not have access to physical therapists' musculoskeletal expertise. I was seen as something of a novelty. Thus began my quest to synthesize a more complete understanding of how dysfunction and injuries were related.

A BREAKTHROUGH

While treating one of these people, Debbie, I had an epiphany. Debbie had a 15-year history of neck pain and migraines after two back-to-back motor vehicle accidents, and she had tried everything and everyone to find relief. After a few sessions, I realized that her problem did not lie in her neck, but in her shoulder. I had made a critical connection that I previously hadn't thought about before: the structural damage the accidents had created wasn't the cause of her pain; it was caused by dysfunctional biomechanics that created vulnerabilities and which the accidents had exacerbated. We addressed these functional issues, and within a few days her pain had disappeared.

Just as I was finishing with Debbie, I discovered a book that confirmed my diagnosis and treatment approach with her as well as a few of my other chronic pain patients. Written by Dr. Shirley A. Sahrmann, a physical therapist out of Washington University in St. Louis, *Diagnosis and Treatment of Movement Impairment Syndromes* is a medical textbook that provided the missing link I had been seeking to pull together my observations. Many of the biomechanical paradigms and rehabilitative exercises in the Fixing You series have been adapted from Dr. Sahrmann's brilliant textbook. I recommend that all physical therapists purchase the book and attend her courses.

Another book I regularly reference is Florence Kendall, Elizabeth McCreary, and Patricia Provance's classic, *Muscles Testing and Function*. This textbook is a wealth of information for understanding precise musculoskeletal anatomy and testing. It is a standard in physical therapy, and I regularly refer to it for isolating muscle testing. It guides me in specifically analyzing and thinking creatively about function. By understanding muscle function on a basic level, I can better hypothesize functional deficits that may be occurring at a systemic level.

But my books are written for laypeople, not medical professionals, to guide you in healing yourself. I've simplified and distilled my medical training to reflect the majority of problems I've found when treating clients. I've prioritized the corrective exercises I've found most powerful for most conditions. I've bolded vocabulary words and added information boxes to help clarify words or concepts. I've also created videos of all the exercises and tests to enhance the effectiveness of your program. To access these free video clips, visit my website **www.FixingYou.net**. Type in the code at the end of this book to access the extra material.

HOLISTIC FUNCTION

The body is the sum of individual units working together to create functional movement. Bones, muscles, tendons, nerves, and ligaments can all be addressed individually, but it is important to understand how these structures work collectively to fulfill a purpose: pain-free movement of the body. So, while it is imperative that individual "chinks in the armor" are found and corrected, visualizing how the whole works together is just as important. This concept also works from the other direction; training movement and/or function reinforces and assists in correcting individual muscles' poor performance. In this book, I've introduced the key individual players—the parts that make up the whole—and also shown how they play together to create function, much like a symphony. You are responsible for bringing them in line to create your concert.

I wish you the best in your pursuit for solutions to your pain. You are not alone in your search for answers. I truly believe that, with a little thought and effort on your part, the Fixing You approach will help you find your answers, as it has for my clients.
The beauty of the body is that results happen quickly when you are doing the right thing. Most of the clients you will read about, and those who aren't included in this book, feel significantly better after only one or two treatments. Often, my clients understand they are on the right path within minutes of performing an exercise. Emboldened by this sense, they become more committed to the process of fixing themselves. You can have the same feeling of empowerment. There is no magical technique or device that will fix you. Only you can fix you—so let's get started on giving you the tools to do just that.

1 | MINDFUL HEALING

There is not a single problem in LIFE
you cannot RESOLVE, *provided you*
first solve it in your INNER WORLD,
its place of origin.

—PARAMAHANSA YOGANANDA

Time and time again I see clients who have tried so many unsuccessful cures that they just don't know what to do. This is worrisome—not because I believe I can't help them, but because they don't believe they can help themselves.

The most powerful aspect of the Fixing You approach is that it shows you what is wrong, actually getting you to feel that certain muscles or movements are not working and how your pain changes when they are corrected. This helps define the problem. It gives issues a beginning and an end, allowing you to compartmentalize pain and therefore see when and how the solution will happen.

Given the tools to understand and correct your injuries, I hope you will feel a sense of empowerment that will motivate you to work harder to fix yourself. If you can define an injury, then you have the power to fix it—and that motivation will get you results.

Getting your head into your plan is essential. Without your commitment, chances are it will never get done. The exercises and techniques I describe in this book will only help you if you commit to them—or more importantly, if you commit to yourself. You cannot pursue any program halfheartedly and expect to get the big payoff. If I find myself more committed than my client, our work is done. I cannot want it more than them. In my experience, there are three processes involved with positive change: You have to visualize the problem and the change needed to solve it, verbalize your intention and write down a plan of action to fix it, and take action to implement your plan.

VISUALIZE THE PROBLEM

Visualization of ideal movement is difficult for many people with chronic pain conditions. This is largely because they are unfamiliar with the anatomy of their injuries or the reasons their injuries exist. The information in this book will help you "see" what's at the bottom of your pain and how to fix it by giving you a glimpse into the underlying anatomy.

You'll notice that as much as I discuss the anatomy of a problem, I also talk about movement. There's little use in learning anatomy if you don't also learn how it creates movement. You will learn what happens to your joints if your muscles are not working correctly and how that causes pain.

This brings me to another reason why visualization can be challenging. Most chronic pain is the result of years of poor movement habits—habits that have taken on the guise of "natural" movement, even though these are actually unnatural and harmful habits (also called movement dysfunctions or movement faults). For instance, you will discover that many people who experience hip or knee pain have pelvic muscles that don't move well. The pelvis houses the muscles that control the hips and knees. When those muscles don't perform well, excessive movement and pain can result. This excessive movement causes pain. Correcting these issues results in patients sensing they are using their leg in a different way—yet it feels better.

> Creating **positive change** involves internalizing your desire, verbalizing your intention, and acting on it.

This tells me that their sense of biomechanically correct movement is actually wrong. What they "visualize" as ideal movement needs to change. To this end, I often ask my clients to perform their exercises in front of a mirror to give feedback on their form. Most people have never taken the time to observe their movement patterns, and this is a real eye-opener for them. You will need to retrain your body's movement habits because chances are that you've been reinforcing your movement dysfunctions for years, if not decades.

In the case of muscles that aren't working correctly, visualize them scrunching up and getting shorter when trying to contract them, and visualize them lengthening when stretching. Tap the muscle briskly to get it to "wake up." As you will see by reading my clients' stories, healing a muscle that has been under chronic

> Set aside 10 seconds throughout the day to **get in touch** with your body and visualize its muscles.

stress can occur almost instantly. The muscles only need to relearn how they should perform. In many cases, pain will instantly diminish or be eliminated altogether.

Look at the illustrations of key muscles in this book, and take some time to visualize where they are on your body and what they do. Using your fingers, feel the area in question to help yourself consciously connect with it. You will need a friend or spouse to help you test your gluteal muscles and pelvic symmetry.

VERBALIZE YOUR INTENTION

Solidify your ideas and support your intention to heal by talking to friends or family or writing down your plan. Often, discussing plans brings their fruition one step closer.

I think all of us have had a time in our lives where we secretly challenged ourselves to reach a goal but didn't tell anyone about it because saying it would heap more responsibility on our shoulders to make it come true. I've run into this situation countless times, where a client won't dare say they expect to become pain free for fear of not meeting their goal and being disappointed. Even when they become pain free, they still doubt that it will continue. Take the plunge and express your goal or desire to eliminate your pain. Put that responsibility on yourself. Hold yourself accountable for following through with this process of fixing your pain. Come up with a short phrase that affirms your intention, and repeat it throughout the day. "Every day, my body is working better and better" is an empowering statement that will help you keep a positive mental attitude. You can make this statement because it is completely realistic, as opposed to setting an unrealistic goal, like running a three-minute mile.

Your body is not designed to be in chronic pain. Something you are doing or not doing is perpetuating your condition. Commit to yourself by telling your friends and family about your goals. By telling friends and family that you believe you will become pain free, you have already made a shift in your consciousness to believe that it will happen. Say it! Your friends and family will probably offer to help you in any way possible. This would be a good time to ask them to help you assess your pelvic symmetry!

Physical therapists use **short- and long-term goals** to create our treatment plans—and you should do the same.

So often in my life, when I'm working toward achieving a goal and getting hung up, I write about what I am doing and the problem I am facing. This small act helps me clarify what I need to do to get from point A to point B. Write down your thoughts and experiences in a journal. Track your progress. If you're getting stuck on a particular concept or exercise, write about it. What is it that you don't understand? Where are you getting stuck? The act of writing will help you see clearly where you are going wrong. It will also help you see what you are doing right and how far you've come since beginning to take action.

Write down how many hours (or minutes) of a particularly painful activity you can do before pain sets in. Write down how many repetitions of an exercise could be completed before you became fatigued. Check your progress in a couple weeks. Can you perform the activity longer before you feel pain? Can you do more repetitions before you experience fatigue? Have you learned a technique that eliminates your pain? Have you uncovered a habit that contributes to your pain?

All of these are great places to begin when tracking your progress. If you did something new that really hurt, then write it down. Figure out why it hurt. Make the necessary adjustments and see if those helped. On the other hand, if you found something that really helped, then write this down as well. It will be valuable information for you to implement later if you hit a plateau.

Create and write down two short-term goals like the following examples: "I will perform my exercises using correct form five times a day for the next week"; "I will set up 10 reminders at work, at home, and in the car to help me change my habits during the next week"; "In the next four days, I will identify 10 circumstances during which I notice my knees excessively rotate inward." Long-term goals should build on your short-term goals, like the following examples: "I will increase my exercise repetitions, using correct form, by 10 repetitions over the next four weeks," or "I will increase my exercise routine to include two strengthening exercises within three weeks."

TAKE ACTION TO IMPLEMENT YOUR PLAN

Finally, you must take action to reach your goals. I guarantee that if you do not take action, your goals will not materialize. So often, I give clients exercises to practice that clearly are instrumental in fixing their pain. When I see them next, however, I frequently find they've only performed one or two exercises since our last visit. This is not the most effective way to address chronic pain.

When you have a chronic pain condition, one repetition of an exercise each day will not fix it. You may initially have to exercise several sessions each day until the length or strength of the involved muscles are at least partially corrected. Once this is accomplished, your pain will diminish, and you can begin whittling down the exercises.

Often, a maintenance plan is necessary because movement dysfunctions are what most likely got you into trouble in the first place. These will be more difficult to identify and correct because they are habits, and habits aren't easily broken. Throughout this book, I've offered some guidance for identifying common movement dysfunctions to help you recognize these and to get you started on correcting them. Ultimately, to permanently eliminate pain, these habits must be corrected.

Bringing your attention to what you are doing will be the most difficult aspect for many of you. In this book, you will find techniques and exercises to ease or eliminate your pain for good. You must, however, feel and notice how your body is moving and performing the exercises. Attending to your specific mechanics will deliver results. I see it all the time, and your body is built no differently than all the other people this approach has worked for.

With the demands of our busy days, it can be difficult to stay focused on these changes. That is why I recommend you set up a way to remind yourself of your new goals and to check in on your habits. Wear a special bracelet, ring, string, or rubber band around your wrist to remind you of the changes you are evoking in your mind and body. Place stickers on the dashboard of your car, the clock, your watch, your telephone—anything you use or look at frequently—to remind yourself that you are getting better every day by correcting those habits that feed your pain.

People often believe that they will have to permanently set aside a lot of time for exercise. Not true. I am asking you to make time over the next two to four weeks to heal yourself. If that doesn't sound realistic to you, then you need to rethink your priority of fixing yourself. Each session should take no longer than five to seven minutes, two to five times each day. In total, I am asking you to take 35 minutes a day for the next two to four weeks to get rid of years worth of pain. That doesn't sound too bad, does it?

THE MIND–BODY CONNECTION

A woman I treated during my first year out of physical therapy school is a great example of how powerful a tool the mind is in affecting our bodies. Iris was one of my first patients. Her diagnosis was intermittent cyanosis, which basically means that her extremities occasionally turned blue due to lack of oxygen.

Now, this isn't something we learn about in physical therapy school, so I took an extensive history that included a husband who had suffered a heart attack and been hospitalized a few months earlier. After this, Iris went home and scrubbed her house from top to bottom. The next morning she awoke with blue fingertips and lips. She went to see doctors, specialists, herbologists, acupuncturists—you name it. No one had a clue as to the solution, and neither did I.

I decided to do some range-of-motion and strength testing. As we began moving, her fingertips, toes, and lips turned blue. As a first year grad, I knew enough to know this wasn't good. So I gave her a few stretches, making sure she understood to stop if anything turned blue, and sent her home. After she left the office, I called the referring doctor.

"I just had Iris in here, and she turned blue during my exam," I began.

"Yes, we've seen that happen too," replied the doctor.

"Have you done blood tests to see whether there is a chemical cause for her symptoms since this seems to correlate to her cleaning episode?" I asked.

"We've run every test we can think of. Nothing abnormal shows up," replied the doctor.

"I've never seen this before," I said.

"Neither have we," said the doctor. "Just do your best. We have to exhaust all avenues, and she's been through just about everything and everyone."

After three days practicing stretches, Iris returned. "Still turning blue," she offered. She was visibly upset. In my mind, I believed there was no exercise I could offer her that would correct this problem. I went back to her history and we talked.

"Iris, your husband had a heart attack three months ago," I began. She nodded, looking concerned.

"How's he doing?"

"He's much better. He's just started a walking program." She brightened a little.

Then what I needed to say next came to me. I looked her straight in the eyes and said, "Iris, your husband isn't going to die." She blinked. "And neither are you," I continued. She blinked again and let out a deep breath.

I felt I was onto the source of her problem and continued,

"Have you ever spoken of this to a therapist, counselor, priest, or friend? Anyone who you can confide in?"

"No, I haven't," she said.

"Then your treatment is to do so within the next four days. I'll see you in a week," I finished.

She came back next week, arm-in-arm with her husband and looking radiant.

"I just wanted my husband to meet you," she said and smiled. "This is him," she told her husband.

"How are you feeling?" I asked hopefully.

"No symptoms at all! Look!" She did all her exercises with no signs of cyanosis.

"Amazing," I said.

"I spoke with a therapist, and I feel so much better! I can do anything!" she exclaimed.

"Yes, you can," I said. We spoke some more and then hugged goodbye.

This has always struck me as a dramatic example of the mind's influence over the body. I cannot explain how her mind affected her blood flow the way it did, but the connection seemed clear. We read stories almost daily in the newspaper about similar phenomena—people holding on to their lives through sheer will after being trapped in an earthquake or becoming elite athletes after conquering a life-threatening illness. We've all read or heard about Eastern mystics able to control almost every aspect of their bodies through meditative practice. Tapping into your brain's power to control your muscles, monitor your habits, or feed your desire to become better will be a large part of you remaining pain free after identifying and fixing the physical issues causing your pain. If Iris can restrict blood flow to her extremities and then reverse it, then surely we can master the way we move and function, and thereby live pain free.

My experience tells me that no matter what diagnosis you have or what kind of accident you were in, the body must learn to move correctly in order for tissues be pain free or to experience significant pain reduction. This book teaches you to assess your movement patterns and correct the most common issues preventing ideal movement.

THE POWER OF WILLPOWER

Some people make goals because they'd like to achieve an end—and some people make goals because they *must* achieve an end. The second group are the people who get the work done, and usually above and beyond what I've asked of them. This is embodied in Ernie's truly inspirational story. Ernie had a traumatic brain injury as a result of being hit by a drunk driver while he was in a bike race. This happened three years earlier, and Ernie wanted to ride in that race again to prove to himself that he could do it. He had been through so much with his rehab, return to work, and family issues. This was one last big hurdle he wanted to clear.

I met Ernie and liked him immediately. I didn't have much experience working with people with brain injuries, just my clinical rotation during physical therapy school. I knew that these people need to limit stimuli (bright lights, loud noises, strength challenges, balance, and so on) because their brains have difficulty filtering the information.

But Ernie had fire in his eyes, and I could see he was committed in spite of his obvious challenges with cognitive, balance, strength, and flexibility deficits. We began by working in a dim, quiet room with no distractions and rigged up a bike with exercise stretch tubes to get him comfortable sitting on a bike again and relearning how to balance himself. I gave him instructions in simple sentences with plenty of time in between for processing. Once we mastered those skills, we moved on to standing balance and strengthening, while learning how Ernie's brain responded to physical exertion and simultaneously receiving instructions. He made excellent progress while we tailored his program to his specific needs.

I had the idea to make a set of training wheels for his transition to the bike outside. I visited several bike shops and spoke to their mechanics about my situation; each one told me to forget it, saying that I'd never get a person with a brain injury to ride a bike because it would be too difficult. That just fired me up even more. "You don't know Ernie," I thought.

Finally, we decided that I'd hold on to the bike while he rode. Ernie was scared at first, and so was I. If a person with a brain injury hits his head, he is more susceptible than the rest of us to further injury. Until that point it was relatively safe, innocuous work with no chance of further injuring his brain. But to achieve Ernie's goal of riding in his race, we had to take some risks. He had worked hard, and it was time to take the next big step.

Ernie and I went out to the parking garage, and he mounted the bike. I held on and ran with him while he pedaled and found his balance. We continued this for many sessions: I gave Ernie instructions, Ernie responded, and both of us learned how far we could push the envelope with this whole new level of difficulty.

Until one day Ernie said, "Let go."

"Are you sure?" I asked, huffing.

"Yes, I can do it. Let go," he answered.

I did. And he did.

He rode like a dream for 10 minutes. Once I saw his telltale signs of mental fatigue it was time to get off. While I held the bike for Ernie to dismount, I looked into his eyes. He was exhilarated and had engaged with plenty of stimuli for the day. Neither of us said a word. The hard work was done—then it was just a matter of building up his endurance.

I had never been as proud of someone as I was of Ernie that day in the garage. He stared down his fears and setbacks and rose above them in spite of all the evidence that he should not have been able to do what he did. He was and is a real hero and inspires me to this day. By the way, he rode in that race and finished, three years after being hit on his bike with only the chin strap of his helmet left intact. There is no reason you cannot achieve similar greatness and pride in your own accomplishments. You just have to begin.

Ernie faced his demons and conquered them. In spite of everything working against him, he drew from his vast inner strength to do what no one else believed he could do. Fixing chronic pain is no different, except with one caveat: Instead of others not believing in you, it is usually you who does not believe in yourself. It's no wonder, after seeing specialists and therapists who couldn't help you or after seeing images of structural damage and being told this was the cause of your pain. This time will be different because you will have the keys to unlock the mysteries of your pain.

ATTENTION AND AWARENESS

Chronic aches and pains aren't just for those who have been involved in accidents. I've found similar biomechanical problems at the roots of chronic pain in people who have had traumatic accidents as well as in those who didn't. Therefore, I believe accidents expose and exacerbate existing vulnerabilities in our bodies. Fixing someone who was involved in a motor vehicle accident that resulted in chronic back pain has been no different than helping someone who has had back pain for decades and has never been involved in an accident. They both require an understanding of how poor function is feeding the problem and what needs to be corrected to eliminate pain. Essentially, in order to fix your body and eliminate chronic pain, you need to pay attention to how your body moves.

I used to work at a health club. While I was in the locker room changing after a workout one day, a man approached me.

"Hey, do you mind taking a look at my arm? I bumped it last week, and now I don't seem to have the strength like I used to," he said.

"Sure," I said.

In three seconds, I knew exactly what his problem was; he had completely severed his biceps tendon at the elbow. His injured arm was visibly smaller than the other, and the biceps muscle was curled up in a little ball up by his shoulder, similar to the way blinds roll up on windows. It was as if someone had stuffed a sock into his upper arm.

> If you are interested in learning more about specific hip or knee diagnoses, go to the WebMD website (www.webmd.com), a good source of medical information. To this end, the Family Doctor website (www. familydoctor.org) also has good information.

"You've ruptured your biceps tendon," I said, "and you need to get an orthopedic surgeon to operate on it immediately."

He returned a few days later. "I saw a surgeon, and he said it wasn't torn," he said.

"Go see another surgeon—it's torn. I guarantee it," I said. "And do it fast!" I added.

I saw him a month later in the locker room. "You were right," he said. "I saw another surgeon, and I had an emergency operation that day."

This man was not in touch with his body. Many of you reading this book are in a similar situation—not ever considering how different parts of your body work together to create pain-free movement. In the above case, a man had suffered a traumatic blow to his arm that caused his problem. In this regard, it was a clear-cut issue that had an easily pinpointed cause. Chronic pain that isn't due to trauma is often caused by a gradual decline in the quality of the body's movements. It is time for you to pay attention to your body, and my sincerest hope is that the information in this book will help you do that. The exercises in this book will help you if you check in with yourself and become aware of your body. Always go back to your form and think about what you are doing. Be present and be attentive—you will be rewarded for it!

PAIN: THE GOOD AND THE BAD

The last item I'd like to address is pain avoidance. It is a natural reaction to avoid a stimulus that is hurting you. The operative premise here is that it is *hurting* you. Quite often I need to educate my clients regarding "good" pain versus "bad" pain. The discomfort of a fatigued muscle feels different than the pain of a muscle strain or **impinged** joint—pain that indicates injury. Learning to tell the difference between "good" pain (the temporary discomfort of retraining your body) and "bad" pain (pain that indicates injury) is important to your healing process.

Generally, what I'm referring to as "good" pain is a feeling of fatigue in the muscles or tissues you are exercising or trying to restore range of motion to. Muscle fatigue may be uncomfortable, but it doesn't mean that what we're doing is hurting us—in fact, that feeling of fatigue lets us know that we are getting stronger. Muscle fatigue also indicates that your body has had enough for the time being. Listen to your body. Stop when you need to. Don't try to push through another set of repetitions or add more weight until your body is ready. Avoiding the message your body is sending doesn't do you any favors and ultimately slows down your progress because ignoring good pain establishes compensatory behavior that can contribute to bad pain.

For example, imagine that you are performing a biceps curl, bending your elbow to bring your hand to the top of your shoulder and then lowering it back down to your side. Weight lifters perform this exercise with weights in their hands to strengthen the biceps muscles in the front of their arms. To maintain good form during this exercise, the arm should stay roughly at the midpoint of the trunk while curling the hand up and down. This helps the head of the arm bone, nestled in the shoulder socket, remain in its proper position with limited stress to the shoulder joint tissues.

Keeping the arm in a mechanically correct position fatigues the biceps muscles more quickly and with lighter weight. However, pushing past fatigue in order to reach a predetermined number of repetitions or lift heavier weight, the elbow compensates by rocking forward and back. When the elbow moves back, the head of the arm bone at the shoulder joint moves forward, often pulling the shoulder blade with it or stressing the tissues in the front of the shoulder. Over time this can create a host of mechanical problems in the shoulder joint.

Biceps fatigue during curls is good pain because it indicates that the muscle is being stimulated to strengthen and grow. This is what we are shooting for when performing the strengthening exercises at the end of this book. We want muscle stimulation and therefore improved strength and control of the bone or joint in question. In the biceps curl example, ignoring this fatigue to squeeze out a few more reps or allow you to lift more weight can cause shoulder joint problems. Become comfortable with and even rejoice in the fact that the muscle you are targeting is fatiguing. It is better to strengthen the muscle group incrementally rather than compensate your form—and your healing process—to squeeze out a few more repetitions. This is where bad pain comes in.

> **Slow down** and feel what your body is telling you when performing the tests and corrective exercises and when you're out and about during the day.

Avoidance of good pain—ignoring your body's signals—often leads to "bad" pain. Bad pain is more difficult to describe because everyone experiences it differently. It can be sharp or dull, nagging or acute. It is the pain you are trying to eliminate, the pain of injury or dysfunction. It is something you feel that you instinctively know shouldn't be happening.

You should only feel fatigue in the muscles you are targeting. Using the biceps curl example, if you feel pain at the shoulder or elbow joints while performing the curl, then you know you're experiencing bad pain. The biceps muscles are located between the shoulder and elbow joints. If you feel pain above or below the biceps muscles, it is likely that you are lifting too heavy a load or allowing your elbows to move too much. The habits that cause bad pain ultimately compromise your efforts, leading to tissue vulnerability and weakness—and more pain.

So often, clients are disappointed to find that they fatigue quickly when exercising with correct form. I happily point out that this is great news because they are finally activating and strengthening the right muscles without exacerbating their condition! Keep this in mind as you strengthen through your injury.

2 UNDERSTANDING YOUR ANATOMY

KNOWLEDGE *of any kind gets metabolized spontaneously and brings about a* CHANGE *in* AWARENESS *from where it is possible to create* NEW REALITIES.

—DEEPAK CHOPRA

Understanding **hip** and knee pain requires a little knowledge of anatomy, biomechanics, and movement. Musculoskeletal pain is often due to three problems that feed each other. There are anatomical changes such as tight or weak muscles. There are biomechanical issues such as whether your leg bone (**femur**) is moving well in the hip socket. And there are movement faults such as poor standing or walking habits. Movement faults reinforce the anatomical issues, which support the biomechanical changes, which help create the movement habits (Figure 2.1). This is a cycle of chronic pain that can happen anywhere in the body. The Fixing You approach addresses problems at all three levels so you can permanently fix your pain, rather than just reduce symptoms.

This book will teach you where most problems occur that cause hip and knee pain. These will probably parallel your problems as well. The underlying issues we'll discuss may manifest as pain in different areas, but the root problems are essentially the same. The reason for this, as you'll soon see, is that muscles controlling the hips and knees have multiple functions. For instance, a muscle that is not performing well may alter how the head of the femur is tracking in the hip socket, or it may allow the thigh bone to rotate too much, causing knee pain.

Chronic Pain Cycle

Figure 2.1 Fixing pain involves correcting each part of the pain cycle.

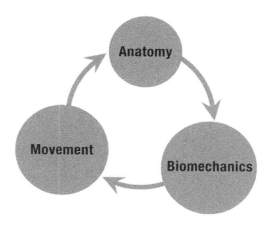

My goal is to introduce you to the major players and show what their jobs are. I'll try to keep the information simple and always try to reorient you back to our pain cycle: anatomical changes cause biomechanical problems, which contribute to movement habits that reinforce the original anatomical and biomechanical problems.

Most hip or knee pain can be distilled down to three problems: poor performance of the muscles in the back of the **pelvis**, overly tight muscles in the front of the pelvis, and poor movement habits that reinforce both these issues. Essentially, hip and knee pain have their roots in poor pelvic muscle performance. If you can keep these three ideas in mind while reading through this book, you'll be way ahead of the class in terms of understanding why you have pain and how to fix it. This includes pain from diagnoses such as **osteoarthritis**, bursitis, **ITB-friction syndrome**, **sciatica**, groin pain, SI joint dysfunction, **patellofemoral syndrome**, chronic hamstring strains, **anterior knee pain syndrome**, and more. These diagnoses describe the structures or tissues that are stressed. Therefore I call them structural diagnoses. These are things that may show up on MRIs or X-rays or fall under headings such as syndromes if there isn't an easy scapegoat to point to. I don't treat structural diagnoses because these tissues are merely responding to adverse stresses caused by other problems.

> A **syndrome** is simply a **group of symptoms that commonly happen together**. A diagnosis of anterior knee pain syndrome (AKPS) means you have pain in the front of the knee, usually when climbing stairs or after sitting for a while.

Instead, I help people correct the underlying issues, or functional problems, that cause the stresses. It's my belief that functional problems create structural problems. But more important, functional problems create pain. These issues often lie in each of the elements of our pain cycle above: anatomy, biomechanics, and movement habits. I've found that correcting functional problems removes pain—regardless of whether or not the structural issue is resolved.

For example, arthritis is a structural problem that shows up on an X-ray and is easy to point to as the source of your pain. But most people don't see specialists because they have arthritis. They go because their hip or knee hurts. But pain can be eliminated in people with arthritis if it's not too advanced. Not by curing their arthritis but by fixing the functional problems that cause their pain. Often these are two separate issues. That's what you will learn in this book.

Focusing only on the structural diagnosis is similar to seeing an X-ray of a broken left thumb and appropriately casting it to heal without realizing that the right hand is continually hitting it with a hammer. Until we can make the right hand stop, the left thumb will continue to be reinjured, if it ever really heals at all. Yes, the broken bone is painful, but the right hand continues to deliver more pain and injury, preventing true healing from occurring. I believe something similar is happening that causes these structural changes and chronic pain in the body—no matter where the pain resides.

Looking Closely at the Pelvis and Its Muscles

Central to our understanding of hip and knee pain is the pelvis and the muscles that attach to it. These muscles control the hip and knee joints. I like to think of the pelvis as three bones: the **sacrum** and two **ilia** (Figure 2.2). Each **ilium** houses the hip socket where the thigh bone (femur) attaches to form the hip joint. The ilia also form a joint with the sacrum called the **SI joint** ("S" for sacrum and "I" for ilium).

An array of hip muscles work in concert not only to stabilize the pelvis and move the leg but also to correctly track the head of the femur in the hip socket and control rotation at the knee. Most problems I see involve weak or poorly timed gluteal muscles (the **gluteus maximus** and **gluteus medius**) together with overly tight muscles in the front of the pelvis and poor movement habits reinforcing these issues. So let's look at these and other muscles to understand where they are, how they're supposed to work, and what typically goes wrong.

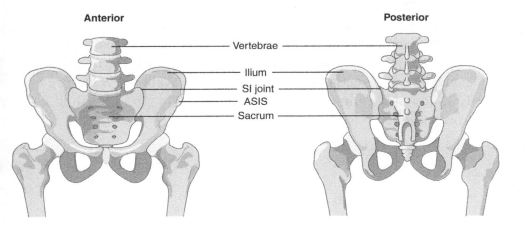

The Pelvis

Figure 2.2 The pelvis is composed of the sacrum and two ilia.

Gluteus Maximus

The gluteus maximus originates at various areas of the sacrum and back of the pelvis. It inserts onto the outside of the femur (Figure 2.3). Most people think of the gluteus maximus as a hip extender (a muscle that brings the leg back behind you), which is correct, but it also has other functions. Namely, this muscle rotates the leg away from you (**external rotation**) as well as assists in stabilizing the head of the femur (**femoral head**) in the hip socket. Correcting these last two functions is often primarily responsible for fixing groin or hip pain. This muscle often becomes weakened due to movement faults such as standing or walking with poor form.

Turning these muscles on and strengthening them can be achieved by correcting walking mechanics (Walk the Walk, page 105) and performing the Gluteal Pumps exercises in Section 3: Corrective Exercises.

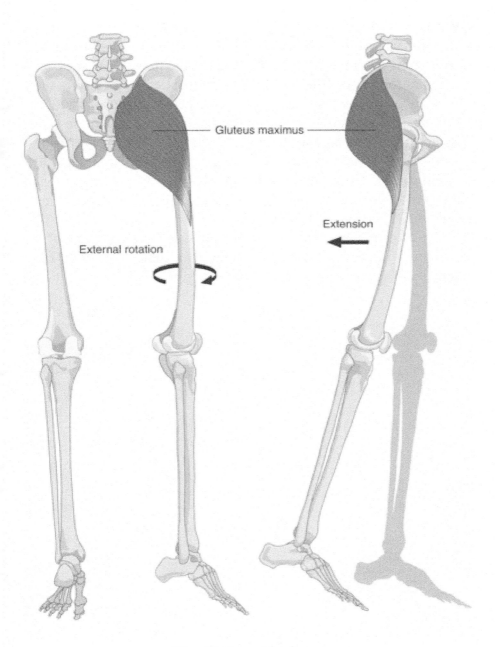

The Gluteus Maximus

Figure 2.3 The gluteus maximus functions to extend and externally rotate the thigh bone. It also helps the head of the femur track properly in the hip socket.

Gluteus Medius

The gluteus medius originates on the top of the pelvis (**iliac crest**), runs from the front to the back of the pelvis, and then inserts into the femur (Figure 2.4). We're most concerned with the portion that comes from the back of the pelvis because it assists with externally rotating and bringing the leg bone out to the side (**abducting**). It also controls how far the pelvis sways from side to side when walking and may help stabilize the femoral head in the hip socket. These actions are important for maintaining the integrity of hip function. This muscle frequently becomes weak due to movement faults.

An effective way of improving gluteus medius function is to perform the Side-Lying Clamshells, Hip Tubes, and Walk the Walk exercises in Section 3: Corrective Exercises.

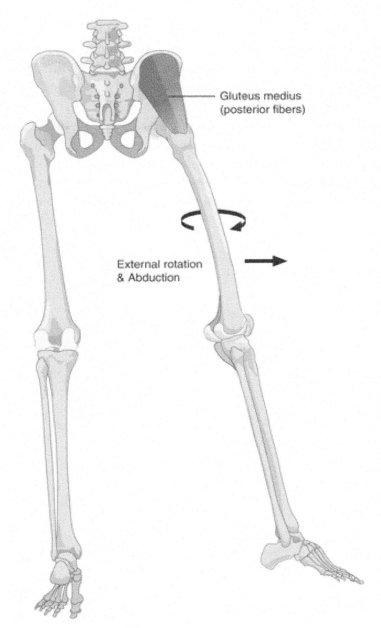

Gluteus medius
(posterior fibers)

External rotation
& Abduction

The Gluteus Medius

Figure 2.4 The gluteus medius functions to abduct and externally rotate the thigh bone. It is also important for maintaining pelvic stability while walking.

Tensor Fascia Lata (TFL)

On the front of the hip is the **tensor fascia lata** (TFL), a relatively small but important muscle that runs from a bony prominence on the ilium called the **ASIS (anterior superior iliac spine)** to a broad band of fascia (**iliotibial band**, or ITB) that inserts into the lower leg bone and kneecap (Figure 2.5). The TFL flexes, rotates inward (**internal rotation**), and abducts the thigh bone, as well as controls the ITB. The TFL can become tight or dominant, which alters pelvic and knee dynamics (discussed in the following).

The TFL & Quadriceps Stretch does a great job of stretching this muscle, and so do the Windshield Wipers exercises in Section 3.

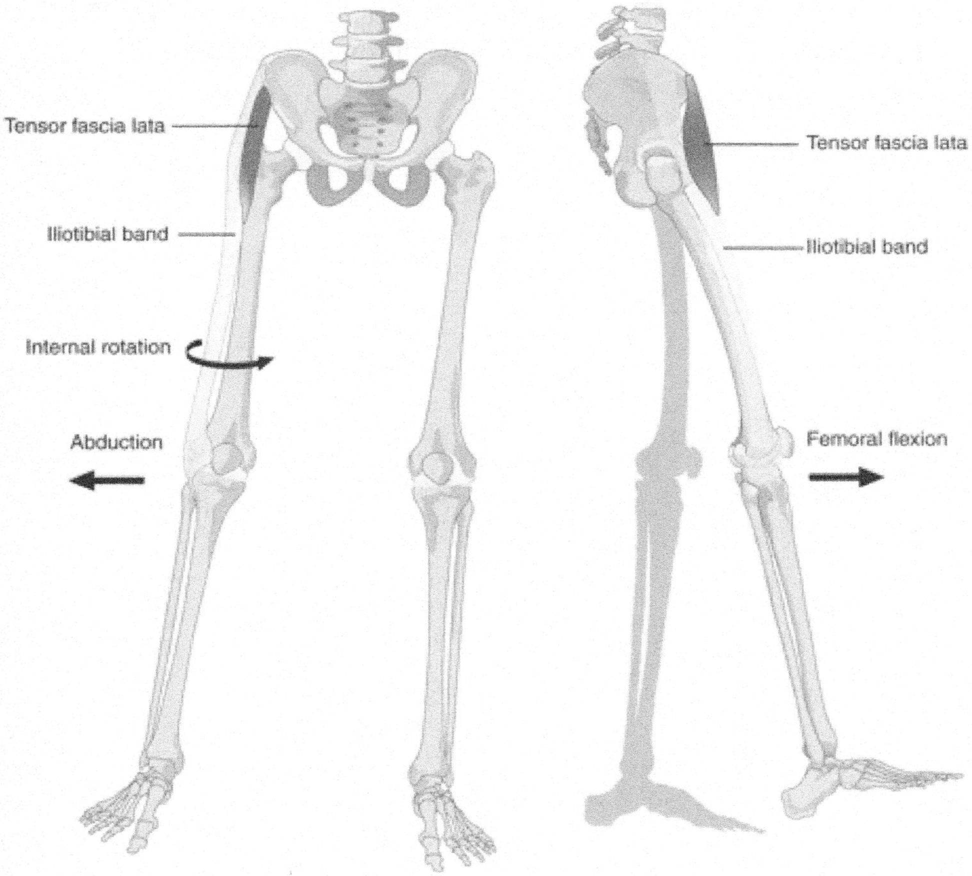

Tensor fascia lata

Iliotibial band

Internal rotation

Abduction

Tensor fascia lata

Iliotibial band

Femoral flexion

The Tensor Fascia Lata (TFL)

Figure 2.5 The tensor fascia lata (TFL) flexes, abducts, and internally rotates the thigh bone.

Iliotibial Band (ITB)

The ITB originates as a deep fascia at the pelvis. It serves as an insertion zone for both the gluteus maximus and TFL, and runs to the outer portion of the top of the lower leg bone, the **tibia**. Although the ITB is not a muscle, it can still affect how the tibia moves. Some fibers blend into the kneecap (**patella**). By virtue of its attachments, the ITB externally rotates the tibia and can influence how the kneecap moves in its groove (Figure 2.6).

Stretching the ITB will not feel the same as if you were stretching, say, the **hamstrings**. It will be more subtle. You can stretch the ITB by practicing the ITB Stretch portion of the TFL & Quadriceps Stretch or the ITB Stretch found in Section 3.

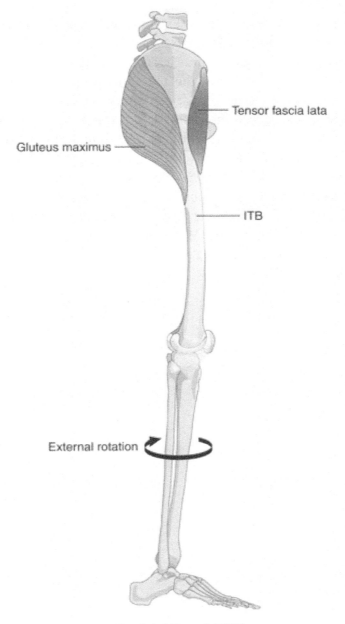

Tensor fascia lata

Gluteus maximus

ITB

External rotation

The Iliotibial Band (ITB)

Figure 2.6 The iliotibial band (ITB) externally rotates the lower leg bone and affects kneecap tracking.

Rectus Femoris

Another muscle that influences how well the pelvis and knee function is the **rectus femoris**—one of the thigh muscles that are also referred to as the **quadriceps** muscles. It crosses the hip joint, originating just below the TFL, and inserts onto the kneecap along with all the other quadriceps muscles (Figure 2.7). When it's tight, it can cause the pelvis to tip forward (**anterior pelvic tilt**), which accentuates the effects of a tight TFL. In addition to knee and hip pain, these muscles are also implicated in back pain (see *Fixing You: Back Pain*). The rectus femoris may also contribute to an abnormal resting position of the kneecap.

Stretching the rectus femoris can be done using the TFL & Quadriceps Stretch and the Windshield Wipers exercises found in Section 3: Corrective Exercises.

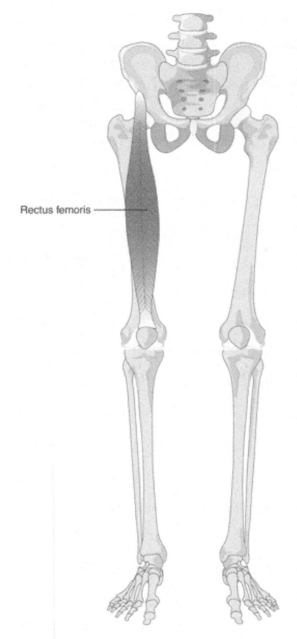

Rectus femoris ⸻

The Rectus Femoris

Figure 2.7 The rectus femoris flexes the hip joint as well as extends the knee joint. It can contribute to a rotated pelvis if tight.

Sartorius

The **sartorius** muscle, like the rectus femoris and TFL, originates at the front of the pelvis and spirals to the inside of the thigh, then inserts onto the upper and inner portion of the lower leg bone (tibia). It flexes, externally rotates, and abducts the hip joint (Figure 2.8). It also helps flex and internally rotate the knee joint.

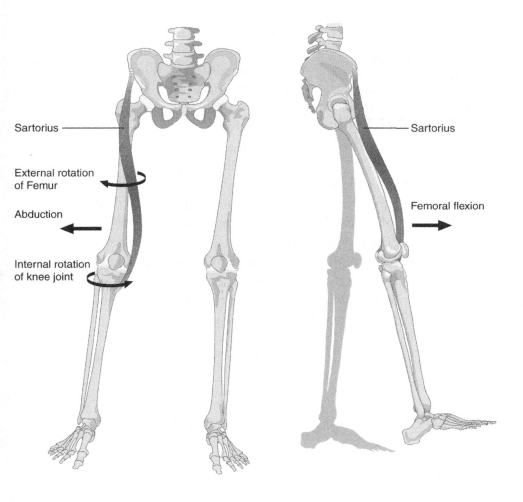

Sartorius

External rotation of Femur

Abduction

Internal rotation of knee joint

Sartorius

Femoral flexion

The Sartorius

Figure 2.8 The sartorius muscle flexes, abducts, and externally rotates the thigh bone. It also contributes to internal rotation of the knee joint, contributing to knee pain.

Hamstring Muscles

On the back of the thigh are the hamstring muscles, which have origins at the back of the ilium as well as on the back of the thigh bone. The hamstrings attach to the lower leg bone and bend the knee joint. They also assist in **extending** the hip. They aren't designed to be the primary hip extensor though, so they don't control the femur head very well. This becomes significant in the presence of weak **gluteals**. When the gluteals are weak, the hamstrings will pick up the slack; this contributes to improper femoral head tracking in the hip socket and, consequently, hip or pelvic pain (Figure 2.9).

> The **hamstring** muscles can become chronically strained or injured due to underuse of the **gluteus maximus and medius.**

Hamstring stretches are ubiquitous in rehabilitation or fitness programs, although I rarely find a need to stretch them except in the case of spinal **flexion** problems leading to back pain (see *Fixing You: Back Pain*). That's why hamstring stretches aren't included in this book; likewise for hamstring strengthening exercises. I rarely encounter hamstrings that are too weak. Instead, I find the hamstrings are typically overrecruited for the reasons we just discussed and are therefore quite strong.

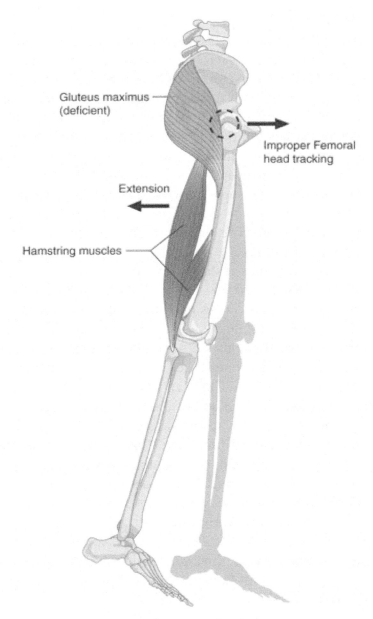

The Hamstrings

Figure 2.9 In the absence of proper gluteal function, the hamstrings become the dominant hip extender and contribute to poor tracking of the head of the femur in the hip socket.

Putting It All Together

We just covered a lot of muscles and leg movements. It's not important that you memorize each one. Just make yourself familiar with the fact that these muscles move both the hip and knee. The muscles often have multiple functions, such as the gluteus maximus, which extends and externally rotates the hip joint as well as guides the femoral head in the hip socket. That's a lot of jobs. So when the gluteus isn't working well, several motions are affected, which can then result in several possible injuries.

You'll also notice that some muscles affect both the upper and lower leg bone movements—sometimes in opposite ways, as in the sartorius muscle, which externally rotates the thigh bone but internally rotates the tibia.

Last, I'd like to point out that many of these muscles overlap in function. For instance the TFL, rectus femoris, and sartorius all flex the hip joint. And the gluteus maximus and part of the gluteus medius both externally rotate the thigh bone. To me, this is important because it shows the body has several redundant muscles for the same job. Therefore if one muscle begins to fail, another can seamlessly take up the load. This can't go on forever though, so problems arise when the backup muscle ends up doing too much of the work for too long (as in the case of the hamstrings overworking due to poor gluteal function). That's why it's important to look at overall function and tease out the players (finding functional problems) rather than just look at one specific tissue that is injured (focusing on structural problems).

Most of what we've covered here falls under the "anatomical" portion of our chronic pain cycle. We've learned where muscles begin and end and what they do. The next section will teach you how biomechanical or movement related problems are created when these muscles aren't functioning well.

Again, don't get caught up in memorizing all these muscles and their functions. Instead, gain an appreciation for the fact the leg and pelvic muscles have multiple functions at different joints.

By the time you finish reading this information, you'll have a decent working knowledge of just what you need to know to fix yourself.

LOOKING CLOSELY AT THE BIG THREE HIP FLEXORS

The TFL, quadriceps, and sartorius muscles comprise what I call the big three hip flexors. These muscles are often overlooked in rehabilitation with more focus placed on a fourth hip flexor, the iliopsoas. In my opinion, though, these three hip flexors cause much more damage due to their size, the fact that they alter pelvic and knee mechanics, and their involvement in just about everything we do with our legs. I think the iliopsoas is usually reacting to these other three hip flexors. I usually don't even address the iliopsoas because its function usually improves once we correct the others' function.

The TFL, rectus femoris, and sartorius muscles often become tight or dominant, especially in the presence of weakened gluteal muscles (gluteus maximus and gluteus medius). The pelvis can develop an anterior pelvic tilt as a result (Figure 2.10).

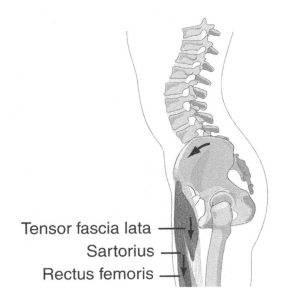

The Big Three Hip Flexors
Figure 2.10 The TFL, sartorius, and rectus femoris attach to the front of the pelvis, potentially tilting it forward into an anterior pelvic tilt.

Tensor fascia lata
Sartorius
Rectus femoris

This can happen on one or both sides of the pelvis. When one side of the pelvis is tilted forward more than the other side, I refer to this as a rotated pelvis. This is discussed in more detail in the section Looking Closely at Pelvic Rotation on page 62. When the pelvic bones become rotated, the muscles controlling hip and knee movements are adversely affected and create pain. This also can appear to be a leg length discrepancy.

Because the TFL controls the ITB, it also influences knee mechanics. A tight ITB will rotate the lower leg outward, which creates stress at the knee joint, especially if the thigh bone is rotated inward. Because the ITB also inserts into the kneecap (patella), it can affect how the kneecap moves when bending and straightening the knee, potentially contributing to AKPS.

Correcting a pelvis that is tilted forward involves strengthening the gluteals (Gluteal Pumps, Walk the Walk, and Side-Lying Clamshells) and stretching the hip flexors in front of the pelvis (TFL & Quadriceps Stretch).

The Gluteals

The gluteus maximus is an important muscle because it is a prime mover of the leg bone into extension (moving the leg backwards) or propelling the body forward as when walking or running. It also helps externally rotate (rotating the leg outward) as previously mentioned. It has another function, though, that's just as important, which is to keep the head of the femur from sliding forward (anterior femoral glide) in the hip socket. If it can't do this, pain results from the femoral head pressing against soft tissues in the front of the hip joint.

The symptoms of a forward-gliding femur can be felt in the front, back, and side of the hip. In the front, groin pain will be felt that may be diagnosed as a tight hip-flexor muscle or groin pull. This also may impinge, or pinch, the **labrum** of the hip socket. However, traditional stretching of the hip flexors will only make the pain worse because this pushes the head of the femur further

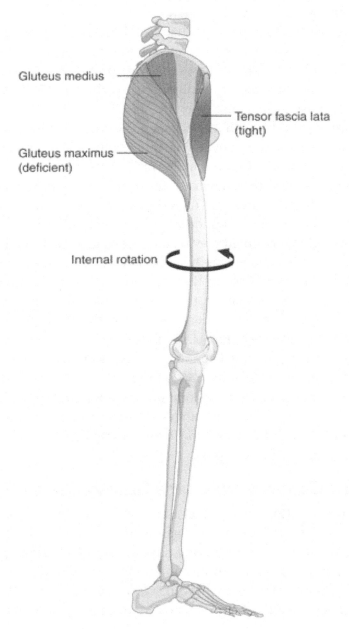

Gluteus medius

Tensor fascia lata
(tight)

Gluteus maximus
(deficient)

Internal rotation

Gluteal Weakness and Femoral Rotation

Figure 2.11 In the presence of weak gluteal muscles, a tight
TFL can excessively internally rotate the femur.

forward, which causes more irritation.

Lateral hip pain may be diagnosed as ITB-friction syndrome or hip bursitis (greater trochanter bursitis) that never seems to heal. It doesn't heal because the root problems—weak gluteus maximus or medius—in addition to overly tight TFL or rectus femoris muscles have not been addressed.

Pain in the back of the hip may be diagnosed as piriformis syndrome that, again, never seems to resolve. The typical answer for these issues is to stretch the piriformis muscle on the back of the pelvis and the hamstring muscles. Although this may feel good, it doesn't solve the underlying problem of dysfunctional gluteal muscles and/or a poorly tracking femoral head.

Last, global hip pain may be diagnosed as an arthritic hip joint. Yes, even arthritic pain can be eliminated using these principles.

A final consequence of the gluteal muscles becoming weak or poorly recruited is that, in the presence of tight hip flexors, the thigh bone will have a tendency to internally rotate too often, too easily, or too much (Figure 2.11, page 53).

You'll soon see this becomes a larger issue with knee pain but can play out as hip pain too. If the femur is held in constant internal rotation, then its axis of rotation will alter slightly while walking and running, which impinges tissues around the socket such as the labrum and a deep hip-flexor muscle, the iliopsoas, which connects to the lumbar spine.

CLIENT CONNECTION: GARY'S GLIDING FEMUR

Gary was an attorney who had a history of arthritic pain in his left hip for five years before we began working together. He had been to see the last of a long line of specialists, all of whom told him that when the pain got to be too much, they would perform surgery for a hip replacement. Well, Gary was 53 years old and far too young to be thinking of that. He was also too young to have this kind of pain for another 10 or 15 years until he had a hip replacement surgery. He was a golfer and basketball player who couldn't get down the court very fast anymore. His golf game suffered due to hip pain that began after the first hole. Even if he did make it through his sports, he couldn't sleep well at night because of pain.

I assessed his hip and found several things wrong. First, he stood asymmetrically, loading one leg more than the other as in figure 2.12 (page 57). This resulted in shortening of some key muscles and lengthening of others. The second problem I found was that the muscles in the back of his pelvis weren't functioning well. As a result, his leg bone (femur) did not rotate or track properly in the hip socket. Instead, it slid forward slightly (anterior femoral glide), which irritated structures in the front of his hip or groin.

The Fixing You Approach for Gary's Hip

Before beginning with corrective exercises, I taught Gary how his habit of standing asymmetrically affected the hip and pelvis. As long as he continued to stand this way, the corrective exercises would not be able to "hold" the fix. This is because Gary would be spending far more time standing and weight-shifting using this pattern than performing the exercises. Poor habits would dominate in the end.

The next step to help Gary was improving range of motion of his hip joint (All-Fours Rocking Stretch). This exercise helped his leg bone move as it should in the hip socket.

Then we stretched the muscles in the front of the pelvis (TFL & Quadriceps Stretch) that contributed to tilting the pelvis forward and overpowered the weaker muscles in the back of the hip. Now the muscles in the back of the hip had a fighting chance to do their job of tracking the femur correctly.

If you have the habit of straightening one or both knees when standing, stick a strip of tape on the back of your locked knee when it is slightly flexed. When you try to lock it again, you'll feel the tape pull, prompting you to unlock the knee.

The final step was to strengthen the muscles in the back of the hip acting on the leg bone (Gluteal Pumps and Walk the Walk). This had a significant effect on his hip pain because the leg bone was no longer sliding forward in the hip socket, impinging tissues such as the labrum and iliopsoas and creating pain.

In the next few weeks, Gary responded well, almost completely eliminating his hip pain for which he was on the verge of a hip replacement. Suddenly he was able to play golf and basketball again and sleep with no pain and full function. His only complaint was that I couldn't help him slam dunk the ball—I'm not a miracle worker!

DAILY HABITS CONTRIBUTING TO POOR MUSCLE FUNCTION

Why do our gluteal muscles become so weak? Why does the TFL become habitually tight? The answer often lies in how we use our bodies. Now we're getting into the "movement habits" part of our chronic pain graphic. As we grow older, we typically look for more energy-efficient ways to do things. Our leg muscles seem to get tired more quickly. One of the easiest things to do to conserve strength and stave off fatigue is to straighten, or "lock," our knees while standing. Doing so allows us to stand on our joints (which possibly contributes to arthritis) instead of using our muscles to hold us up. When we lock our knees to stand, the thigh, hamstring, and gluteal muscles don't need to turn on. Do this often enough and they forget how to turn on. Pretty soon we even develop the ability to walk or run while keeping these muscles, usually the gluteals, turned off.

A variation of this habit is weight-shifting to one leg when standing. We often unconsciously choose one leg to shift to. Let's use the left leg as an example. When you shift your weight to the left leg, the left knee then locks into extension so none of your muscles are being used. The right knee typically flexes and rotates inward in response to this shift (Figure 2.12). This is exactly what the TFL muscle does at the hip joint, so now that muscle shortens, as does the rectus femoris and sartorius muscles. This becomes a chronic condition wherein these muscles on the right side become short while the muscles on the left side remain longer.

Now when the right knee straightens, the tight TFL, rectus, and sartorius muscles pull the right side of the pelvis forward. This creates a rotated pelvis, which we'll discuss later. This is essentially how these movement faults begin, as innocent little rest breaks for the muscles. Then they become habits that create muscle imbalances that either slowly erode our tissues or are ticking time bombs of injury.

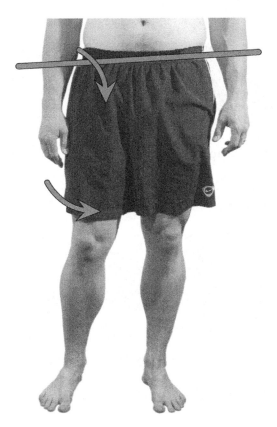

Standing while Weight Shifting

Figure 2.12 This man habitually stands with his left knee locked. This ultimately contributes to a rotated pelvis on one side.

GAUGING YOUR GLUTEALS

We've talked a lot about the gluteal muscles, so now it's time to test yours to see if they're working. You'll need a partner, preferably a physical therapist, to help you. Since most hip problems I see revolve around the gluteus maximus function, or lack thereof, let's start there. This test can be viewed on the Fixing You website at **www.FixingYou.net** after typing in the code at the end of this book.

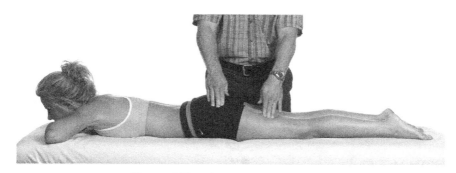

Gluteal Testing, start position

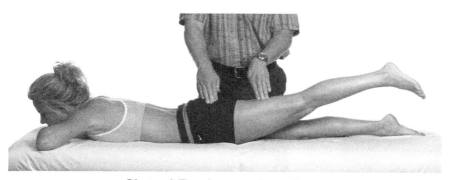

Gluteal Testing, end position

Figure 2.13 Testing the timing of the gluteals versus the hamstrings is important to understanding how gluteal function affects injuries.

First, lie down on your stomach with legs extended. Have your friend put one hand firmly on the gluteals and one hand firmly on the hamstrings. Now raise your leg straight up (Figure 2.13). You will notice the muscles jump (or contract) when testing. Which muscles fire first, the hamstrings or the gluteal muscles?

Chances are it was the hamstrings. The gluteals should either turn on first or at least close to the same time as the hamstrings. Now check the other side. What are the results? Now try to contract the gluteus muscles first. Is it easy or difficult?

Next, while still lying on your stomach, squeeze both rear cheeks together. Does one feel more firm than the other? Does one lag a little prior to reaching its full contraction? Does your back arch in order to squeeze the gluteals? Is one side larger than the other?

Last, still lying on your stomach, bend your knee then lift your leg off the table. Is this easy or difficult? Are you using your hamstrings to do this? Does this hurt your back? Have your friend push down on the thigh. Does it fall easily? If any of these issues is happening, then your gluteals could be weak, an indication of poor gluteus function. Gluteal Pumps and Walk the Walk can help with this weakness.

Walk the Walk: Engaging the Gluteals

Let's look at the gluteals again, this time in a more functional way. Stand up and put each hand firmly on your rear-end muscles. Now walk. Do you feel your gluteal muscles firing? No? You're not alone!

In order to turn them on, you'll first need to know what the gluteal contraction should feel like, so stand still with the left foot forward and the right foot back. Keep your hand on your right gluteals. Contract your right gluteals. Feel them jump in your hand and feel the strength of the contraction. The strength of that contraction should be similar to what's happening when you're walking correctly.

Now relax the glutes and take a step forward with your right foot with your hand still on the right gluteals. When your foot hits the ground, you should feel the gluteus muscles fire almost as strongly as when the right foot was behind you and you consciously turned them on (Figure 2.14). Keep walking and see if that muscle is turning on. Most people will find it is not. It should contract as a consequence of walking correctly instead of from consciously

Walk the Walk

Figure 2.14 Walking to engage the gluteals is a very effective method of re-training these muscles. At foot strike, the knee should be slightly bent with the hips over the foot to best engage the gluteal muscles.

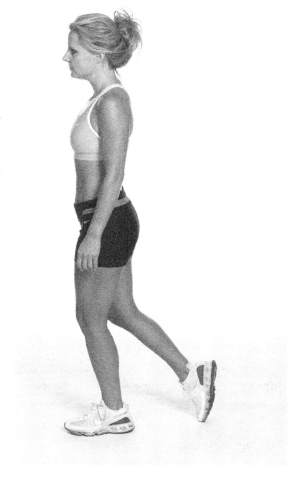

squeezing the muscles. Now check the left. Usually both are not working well, but one is worse than the other. This asymmetry can lead to a rotated pelvis (mentioned earlier).

To correct this, shorten the length of your step so that when your foot strikes the ground, you are striking less through the heel and more through your midfoot or forefoot. Unlock the right knee prior to striking the foot down onto the floor. Make sure the hips are over the foot at footstrike, not behind it. This is the most common movement fault I see with walking—that the hips are too far behind the foot instead of over it. When the body is over the foot (weight-bearing through the arch) and the knee is unlocked at foot strike, the gluteals should naturally turn on. If they do not, then there are three possible causes:

1) The hip is still too far behind the foot.

2) The knee is not unlocked.

3) You are not weight-bearing through your arch.

Lean your hips forward over the knee to engage the gluteus muscles. Now do you feel them? Bend the knee further, maintaining weight through the arch of the foot or bend forward at the hip to get them to turn on. Try this on the other side too.

To retrain the gluteals, you may need to assume a completely exaggerated walking pattern as described above until you become efficient at turning them on while walking. With practice this can happen within a day.

"People will stare at me like this!" some clients complain.

"Only if you keep your hands on your rear like that," I joke.

What feels so unnatural is closer to how you should actually be walking. Your natural walk isn't working anymore. Change is necessary to activate the muscles correctly and start feeding the hip and knee. Gradually your walk will look very similar to how it did before, but with the glutes turning on.

> To check whether your hip is over your foot at foot strike, lift your opposite foot off the ground. If your hips shift forward while doing this, then they are still lagging behind your foot when it strikes the ground.

Until then, you will go through a self-conscious, awkward stage while activating the correct muscles.

"I felt so weird walking like this initially," Susan told me when she began changing her walk. "I thought everyone was staring at me. But now it feels fine. And my hip doesn't hurt anymore."

Susan came to me with hip pain so great she could barely walk and was in tears. After one session of correcting her biomechanics using the principles in this book, she went home feeling 75 percent better. Soon she was completely pain free and progressing her strengthening and cardio training to lose weight and tone her body.

To sum up this section, the gluteals are very important for proper (and therefore pain-free) hip and knee function. Testing the glutes using the exercises above will give you an idea of how well they are working. You can strengthen them using exercises such as Gluteal Pumps but fixing how you stand and walk will have an even bigger impact—especially if you take 10,000 steps each day (recommended for exercise and weight control). So, if you can fix your walk you'll be giving yourself a 10,000 repetition workout without even thinking about it. Talk about buns of steel!

LOOKING CLOSELY AT PELVIC ROTATION

We touched briefly on pelvic rotation so let's look at this idea a little more closely here. Often clients will present with a pelvis where one side is higher or rotated forward more than the other. Although this is often dismissed as a difference in leg lengths, true differences in leg lengths are rare. Typically, the cause is a muscle imbalance pulling on one side of the pelvis in relation to the other. This makes it appear that one leg is longer than the other. It also contributes to a rotated spine and back pain (see *Fixing You: Back Pain*).

There are several muscles attaching to the front of the pelvis which can potentially alter pelvic alignment (Figure 2.15). They are the TFL, rectus femoris, and sartorius muscles.

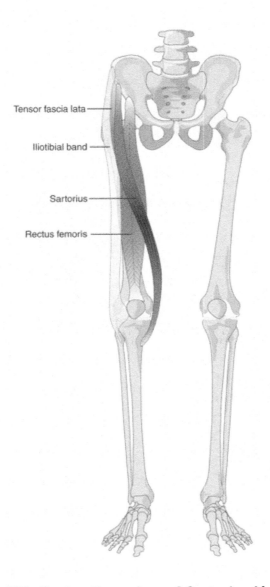

Tensor fascia lata

Iliotibial band

Sartorius

Rectus femoris

The TFL, Rectus Femoris, and Sartorius Muscles

Figure 2.15 The TFL, rectus femoris, and sartorius muscles attach to the front of the pelvis, contributing to pelvic or knee alignment issues.

Earlier I mentioned that poor habits, i.e., standing asymmetrically, can cause one side of the pelvis to develop tighter muscles than the other side. This pulls that side of the pelvis forward and down, creating a rotated pelvis. Pelvic rotation can create height differences between the two hips (Figure 2.16).

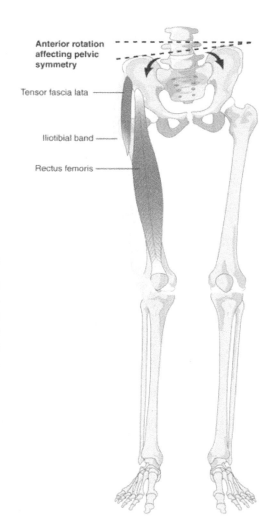

Anterior rotation
affecting pelvic
symmetry

Tensor fascia lata

Iliotibial band

Rectus femoris

The Cause of
Pelvic Rotation
Figure 2.16 Asymmetrical forces acting on the pelvis can create pelvic rotation or relative hip height differences.

Another contributor could be an overly pronated (flat) foot. A pronated foot can functionally shorten a limb relative to the other leg (Figure 2.17). I'd say in about 85 percent of the cases I see, pelvic and knee pain is fixed by addressing the pelvic muscles, not the foot. If pain still persists after correcting hip and knee function, then I consider correcting the foot (see *Fixing You: Foot & Ankle Pain*) including foot orthoses as a last resort.

Pelvic Rotation and Foot Pronation

Figure 2.17 An overly pronated foot can contribute to height differences between two sides of a pelvis.

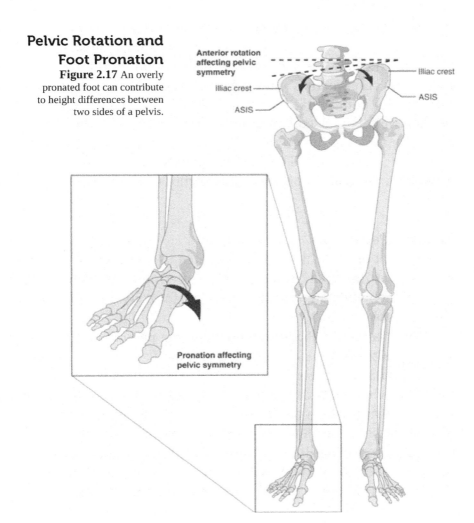

A pronated foot is one whose arch has dropped closer to the floor and contributes to the appearance of a shortened leg. A supinated foot has a higher arch and the opposite effect on leg length appearance.

Both of these scenarios, asymmetrically tight hip flexor muscles and/or a relatively pronated foot on one side, can create the illusion of a leg length discrepancy. Often leg length discrepancies are treated by placing a heel lift in one shoe or by fitting for a pair of shoe inserts (foot orthoses). However, if the true nature of the discrepancy isn't discovered knee, hip, and back pain issues will most likely arise later.

In most cases the main villain here would be the tight hip flexors in combination with weak gluteal muscles. Again reinforced by poor walking, sitting, or standing habits. Correcting this involves a combination of stretching the hip flexors and strengthening the gluteal muscles to restore balance to hip and pelvic mechanics. The TFL & Quadriceps Stretch exercise as well as Gluteal Pumps and Side-Lying Clamshells can help with this.

SI Joint Pain

The SI joint or sacro-iliac joint is located in the pelvis where the sacrum and ilia meet. Many people suffering from pain in the back of the pelvis are told they have **SI joint dysfunction**. But what does this mean?

Now that you've been introduced to the pelvic muscles, you probably already have a good idea of what is causing problems at this joint. You guessed it—the TFL, rectus femoris, and sartorius muscles. They can become tight and rotate one side of the pelvis forward, which can cause shear at the SI joint. This happens because these three muscles are attached onto the ilium, not the sacrum. The ilium rotates forward a little more than the sacrum, which twists the SI joint. A relatively pronated foot may also be contributing to these issues, although this is rare.

Correcting this tightness using the TFL & Quadriceps Stretch together with gluteal strengthening (Gluteal Pumps, Walk the Walk, and Side-Lying Clamshells) usually restores proper balance to the pelvis and does the trick for most people.

CLIENT CONNECTION: LARA'S LAGGING LEFT LEG

Lara was training for a marathon. She was turning 46 and wanted to celebrate in style by proving she was better than ever. Except she wasn't. Even though she had a toned body a 20-year-old would envy, her left leg began to drag at approximately mile 15, and she had pain in the front of her hip that prevented her from running further. She also had knee pain in both knees, which she iced to take the edge off. She noticed that after running, she was barely able to bend forward due to chronic hamstring tightness.

Our exam revealed poor tracking of the leg bone in her hip socket (anterior femoral glide). Her pelvis was also tilted forward (anterior pelvic tilt); this contributed to her hamstring strain and leg dragging. An anteriorly tilted pelvis increases strain to the hamstrings because this muscle group attaches to the pelvis. If the pelvis is rotated forward, then the hamstrings are consequently stretched. If the gluteal muscles aren't working and the hamstring muscles are overworking in a lengthened position, then chronic hamstring strains and tightness results.

We addressed the strength and range-of-motion issues that led to these problems, and she was better within a week. Not only was her foot not dragging, but her hamstrings "miraculously" remained loose during and after her long runs.

The Fixing You Approach for Gluteal Strengthening

Lara's leg dragged because the muscles in the back of the pelvis (the gluteals) couldn't control her femur, which then slid forward in the hip socket. This pressed on one of her hip flexor muscles, the iliopsoas, and caused pain. When muscles experience pain, they tend to shut down. That's why she couldn't lift her left leg anymore.

Her hamstring muscles in the back of her legs were chronically tight because they were doing the work of the deficient gluteal muscles. They were also lengthened too much due to her anterior pelvic tilt. When certain muscles are asked to do too much, they become strained and tight. This is why Lara could barely bend over after her long runs: her hamstring muscles were strained and pumped up and couldn't lengthen until they had a chance to rest.

Lara was very fit and aware of her body mechanics, so she responded quickly to her therapy. Within a week, she had learned to run while activating the gluteal muscles. A big part of this was shortening her stride length to reduce the continual stretch and strain on her hamstrings. The result was no more lagging leg, even after 26 miles, and she could immediately bend down to touch her toes once her hamstrings weren't so fired up.

We achieved this using the same principles outlined earlier in Gary's case.

The TFL & Quadriceps Stretch corrected her rotated pelvis. This allowed symmetrical forces to act through her pelvis and gave the gluteals a chance to do their job.

Gluteal Pumps and Walk the Walk turned on her all-important gluteal muscles. We taught her how to walk and then run properly to keep them activated and tracking her leg bone correctly.

Because Lara had good range of motion in her hip, the Windshield Wipers did not play a large role in her rehab. This is not often the case—especially in runners.

Testing for Pelvic Rotation

We've been talking a lot about a rotated pelvis, so how can you figure out whether yours is rotated? Fortunately, there are easy tests to understand how the pelvis is working. It's better to have someone such as a physical therapist look at your pelvis for you because you won't be able to assess this yourself.

1. Standing on a level surface with both knees straight, have a friend or physical therapist kneel down with both hands on the tops of your pelvic bones (iliac crests) as in Figure 2.18. Look to see whether one side is higher than the other. Differences of 1/4 inch or greater can indicate a pelvic anomaly.

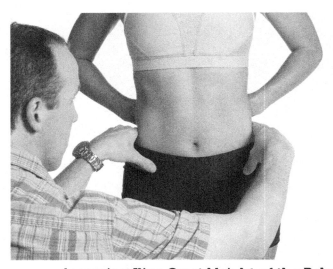

Assessing Iliac Crest Height of the Pelvis

Figure 2.18 Placing fingers on the tops of the iliac crests helps assess whether one side is higher than the other.

2. Now slide the thumbs down and forward until you find a prominent bony ridge on the front of the pelvis. These are the ASISs (anterior superior iliac spines). Keep sliding the thumbs over the ASISs until they just drop off into a more fleshy part of the hip. Stop when you reach this edge of the ASIS and assess the height difference (Figure 2.19). Usually, if one iliac crest is high, then the opposite ASIS will be low. Again, keep your eyes at the level of the pelvis to get a good look. To help you visualize what you are feeling, refer to Figure 2.20.

It is possible that both sides are equally tight and contributing to pelvic problems. Just to be safe, perform the TFL & Quadriceps Stretch even if you don't notice a difference between the right and left sides of the pelvis.

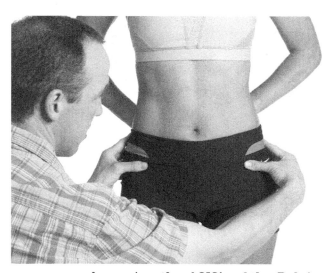

Assessing the ASIS's of the Pelvis
Figure 2.19 Assessing the ASIS of the pelvis gives more information about possible pelvic rotation contributing to hip and knee pain.

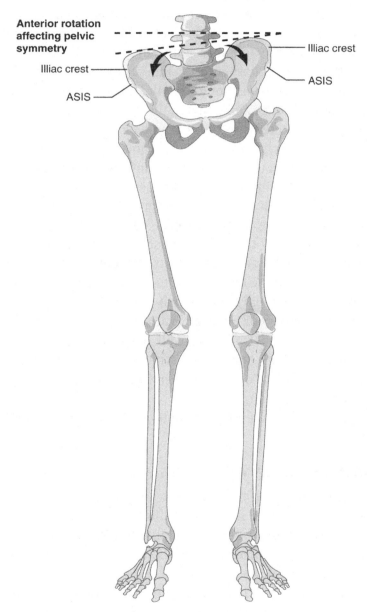

Anterior rotation affecting pelvic symmetry

Illiac crest

Illiac crest

ASIS

ASIS

Pelvic Landmarks

Figure 2.20 Assessing the bony landmarks of the pelvis gives important information about the stresses acting on the hips and back.

Putting It All Together

Okay, let's summarize here for a second. Basically, we've learned that there are three key muscles in the front of the pelvis that can wreak havoc on hip and knee joint function. That terrible triad includes the TFL, rectus femoris, and sartorius muscles. They can be symmetrically or asymmetrically tight, which can create different kinds of aches and pains in the hips or pelvis.

To put this in terms of our chronic pain cycle, tight muscles in the front of the pelvis (anatomical change) can lead to poor tracking of the femur in the hip socket (biomechanical problem), which are reinforced during poor standing or walking habits we've developed (movement faults), which turn off our leg muscles. Turning on one of these muscle groups, the gluteals, can help offset problems caused by those three muscles and eliminate pain.

You've also learned how to assess your gluteal muscles and pelvis (with someone else's help) to determine whether your muscles are strong enough or if the pelvis is rotated. You've also been shown how to fix your walk, activating the gluteal muscles, to improve hip joint mechanics as well as prevent excessive inward rotation of the thigh bone. Correcting this rotation using the exercises in Section 3: Corrective Exercises will be critical to reduce or eliminate your pain.

Okay, now on to a tougher section. You're almost there—stick with me!

LOOKING CLOSELY AT THE LEG

Just when you thought it couldn't get any more difficult, I have to throw in one more issue that I think is important for you to be aware of. Although you won't be able to test this on yourself, it's important to know that our thigh bones can become more or less twisted as we grow.

Have you ever watched a toddler run and noticed how much their feet point inward? That's because babies are born with femurs that are rotated inward (**femoral anteversion**). As they grow and use their legs for running and jumping, the femur untwists to a normal position. Often the femur doesn't untwist enough, which creates an anteverted femur; and sometimes it unwinds too much, which creates a retroverted femur (Figure 2.21). These are impressive words, but don't be scared. They only mean the femur is rotat-

> **Femoral retroversion** and **femoral anteversion** are common structural variances in the rotation of the thigh bone that affect hip, knee, ankle, and foot mechanics.

ed inward (**anteversion**) or rotated outward (**retroversion**). This isn't something we can change, but knowledge of it can help us reduce damage to our hips and knees.

Femoral Retroversion

The figure on page 74 (Figure 2.21) shows a normal and then an outward rotated leg bone (**femoral retroversion**). When a leg bone is rotated out like this, the feet will usually have to follow by pointing slightly outward too. If instead the feet point straight ahead (which we are all taught to do when walking and running), then adverse stresses will be placed on the knee or hip joints. This is because we are trying to override a normal biomechanical condition with our socialized expectations of having feet that nicely face forward.

It's anyone's guess as to whether pain will be felt in the hip or knee under these conditions. That's because pain will happen at whichever joint is able to move the most. Therefore those tissues will be stressed the most. The joint that moves the least will be less affected because it's sitting pretty, right were it wants to be. This is similar to repeatedly bending a copper pipe: eventually, a crease will form at one point, and that's where it will break because the point that moves too much weakens. Every joint in the body works the same way.

So, in the case of a retroverted femur, the feet or knees should point slightly outward to limit stress to the hip and knee joints.

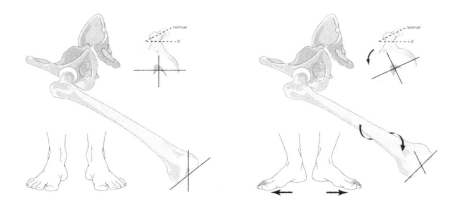

Femoral Retroversion

Figure 2.21 The end of the femur is usually slightly twisted in relation to the head of the femur, as shown in the "normal" image on the left. Variability in the amount of twisting is common, which creates retroversion of the leg bone where the end of the femur is rotated outward, as shown in the "retroversion" image on the right.

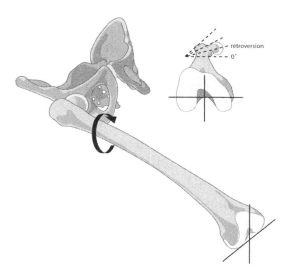

Hip Compensation with Femoral Retroversion

Figure 2.22 With femoral retroversion, if the knee isn't permitted to turn out slightly, the head of the femur sitting in the hip socket will compensate by internally rotating, creating increased stress in the hip socket or knee joint.

This condition is most commonly found in men. This is important because if the knee points straight ahead, then the head of the femur doesn't sit ideally in the hip socket and can cause problems (Figure 2.22) such as groin pain, deep joint pain, or potential structural changes such as arthritis or labrum tears.

In Gary's case, every time he tried to point his knee or foot forward, such as when running or lining up for a tee shot, he was actually rotating the head of his thigh bone deeper into the hip socket, increasing hip joint compression and causing pain.

So we corrected his concept of ideal movement. In terms of his golf swing, it meant allowing his knee to rotate out during set-up. During basketball, we had the same philosophy: allow the knees to slightly rotate out while running. We also changed how he pivoted on his left leg for a lay-up to decrease the internal rotation his hip experienced. This unloaded the compression in the hip socket and eliminated his pain.

Femoral Anteversion

The opposite of retroversion is anteversion: when the femur is twisted inward, although the femoral head sits in the hip socket as it should (Figure 2.23, page 76). This most often happens in females. This might help explain the high incidence of knee injuries in female athletes. Knee injuries in this group usually result from a rotation problem where the lower leg bones twist in relation to the femur. **Anterior cruciate ligament** (ACL) and meniscus tears fall into this category.

Determining whether anteversion exists is important to establish treatment and corrective exercises to reduce compression in the hip or knee joints. With anteversion, if the is leg bone is rotated outward (as when the feet point straight ahead), increased stress is placed on the hip or knee joint (Figure 2.24, page 76). Female joints tend to be a little looser than males', so the propensity for injury is greater. Remember, injuries tend to happen at joints that move too much.

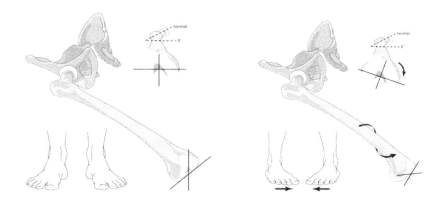

Femoral Anteversion

Figure 2.23 Anteversion is a common structural variance where the end of the femur is rotated inward favoring more of a knock-knee posture, as in the "anteversion" picture on the right.

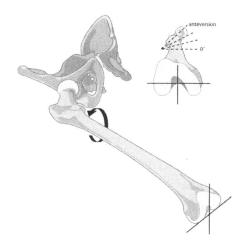

Hip Compensation with Femoral Anteversion

Figure 2.24 With femoral anteversion, if the knee isn't permitted to turn in slightly, the head of the femur will create stress in hip socket or knee pain may be felt.

Tests to determine whether retroversion or anteversion exist can be performed by a physical therapist or assessed via X-ray. Based on these findings, adjusting corrective exercises would be appropriate to maximize benefits. Also, application of this knowledge to sport performance could reduce injuries and improve your competitive edge. While you train or participate in sports, knowing if your femurs are twisted outward or inward will help reduce cumulative stress to your joints.

Well, you've just covered the most difficult concept in this book—that sometimes our thigh bones are more or less twisted than the norm. If one or both are twisted inward, then the hips, knees, and feet do better when the hip external rotators (gluteus maximus and gluteus medius) are strong and control the inward movement well. This should become an important part of your strengthening program. If one or both femurs are twisted outward, then slightly pointing the feet, knees, and hips outward reduces wear and tear to the hip and knee joints. Again, strengthening the gluteals will be important to control rotation of the femurs. It's pretty simple when you think about it.

Hamstring Strains

Before we tackle knee pain I'd like to talk about another common injury I see: chronic hamstring strains. This injury happens most often in runners or cyclists. It can also be diagnosed as **ischial tuberosity pain syndrome** or even ischial tuberosity bursitis. If you remember, the hamstring muscles originate on the ilium of the pelvis. Well, the name of the bony part where they originate is called the ischial tuberosity. I lump these diagnoses together because they all essentially involve the same problem, that of an overly stressed hamstring muscle that either hurts at the belly of the hamstring or where it attaches to the pelvis.

Most people will experience this issue during long runs or rides. They'll also feel burning or intense pain where their rear-end meets the chair when sitting down for more than a few minutes. That's because they're sitting on an irritated muscle. But it's not the sitting that's causing the problem, it's everything else they're doing before and after sitting that's the problem.

I believe it stems from overrecruitment of the hamstring muscles while they are excessively lengthened. Runners try to run fast—after all, isn't that the point? Well, people with chronic hamstring strains try to run fast by lengthening their stride more and pulling through the leg. When the leg is outstretched in front and making contact with the ground, the heel is making most of the contact. This means the hamstring must pull the body over the leg and do so when the hamstring is at its longest, and therefore weakest, position. If you think about it though, the leg can only be so long, so the only way to go faster in this scenario is by pulling harder through the hamstring.

In cycling this may happen if the heel is dropped down during the pulling phase of cycling. When the heel is dropped down, the hamstring is once again maximally lengthened at the moment it is being called on to work its hardest.

In both these scenarios, the functional problem is that the gluteal muscles are not participating enough and instead are letting the hamstrings do all the work. The gluteal muscles help propel us forward when running and help drive the legs while cycling. These athletes must change their form to recruit the gluteals and de-emphasize the hamstrings.

When running, this happens when the stride length is actually shortened, allowing the pelvis to be over the foot at foot strike. This immediately activates the gluteal muscles for propulsion. At the foot level, the foot strike should be less of a heel strike and more of a midfoot or forefoot strike. This turns on a large group of foot and lower leg muscles (see *Fixing You: Foot & Ankle Pain*) as well as more strongly activates the gluteal muscles. It also helps the hamstrings turn off. Remember Lara's lagging leg? Her hamstrings were doing too much of the work. When she shifted her running form to emphasize gluteal function, she eliminated her chronic hamstring fatigue, soreness, and tightness. So the trick is to take shorter steps to turn on the gluteals, and then in order to run faster, you just increase your RPMs (revolutions per minute) instead of your stride length.

Think about it: your stride length is finite, but your RPMs can be trained to increase. It makes more sense to work on moving the legs faster rather than try to reach out farther with the foot and pull harder. When explaining this, I always bring up the vision of Lance Armstrong cruising up the Pyrenees mountains during the Tour de France, passing all his competitors who were using brute strength to try to beat him while he used RPMs. His legs were moving so much faster than his opponents because he's learned that he has only so much strength to pump those pedals—but he has a much higher ceiling on his ability to increase his RPMs. The same goes for running. Shorten the stride and improve the foot strike to activate the right muscles, then increase your RPMs without increasing your stride length. You'll feel like you're floating!

Looking Closely at Knee Pain

Okay, we've talked a lot about the hip joint, the muscles affecting it, and the fact that our femurs may be twisted, which can contribute to hip or knee pain. Let's finally focus on knee pain and understand how all these players contribute to knee function.

The knee joint is deceptively simple. At first glance, it appears its only job is to bend and straighten. How hard can that be? To truly understand this joint, however, it's important to understand that the end of the thigh bone (femur) is irregularly shaped. This shape dictates that if the lower leg is fixed (for instance, when the foot is in contact with the ground), then the femur must rotate inward as the knee joint bends (flexes) and outward as it straightens (extends). If the lower leg is not fixed on the ground (as when kicking a soccer ball), the lower leg usually rotates instead.

This little bit of rotation is where the knee gets into trouble because the large muscles on the front and back of the thigh bend and straighten the knee well, but they are not designed to adequately control knee joint rotation. Instead, the joint surface, meniscus, and **ligaments** guide rotation.

Here's the important part. Remember when I said the femur rotates inward if the lower leg is fixed as in running or walking? Well, most of the muscles that control that rotation are found in the pelvis, not in the knee. They're all the muscles you learned about earlier. Therefore, correcting strength and range-of-motion problems at the hip benefits the knees because these muscles control the femur, which then helps control the knee. The only difference is that more attention should be paid to how the knee is moving.

> **Reminders,** like stickers placed strategically so you'll see them, are a great way to continually **correct movement habits** contributing to pain.

What I mean by this is most knee pain stems from the knee excessively rotating or collapsing in when walking, sitting, or standing. When the knee collapses in, the thigh bone rotates inward (internal rotation). This is stressful to the knee joint tissues. Observing this and preventing it, together with correcting pelvic muscle weaknesses or range-of-motion issues will fix most knee pain. The muscles to target are the external rotators of the leg we discussed earlier, the gluteus maximus and gluteus medius.

Sometimes the foot and ankle can affect knee pain as well. If the foot is overly flat or pronated, this contributes to internal rotation of the lower leg and knee. In my experience, 85 percent of the people with knee pain benefit more from strengthening hip muscles rather than using foot orthoses (shoe inserts) to affect the knee.

A history of ankle sprains can also affect knee pain. This happens as a result of protecting the ankle or if the ankle lacks range of motion. The knee then often makes up for this lack of motion, causing pain.

Let's also not forget our old friends, the big three hip flexors. Due to it's insertion at the inner tibia, the sartorius produces excessive internal twisting of the tibia, which creates stress and pain. The TFL, if you remember, is an internal rotator of the leg bone, which contributes to the excessive inward rotation at the knee joint. One of the best ways to stretch both of these muscles is performing the TFL & Quadriceps Stretch. If this stretch causes knee pain, then allow the thigh to scoot to the outside of the hip joint. This decreases the intensity of the stretch and eliminates knee pain during the stretch. As the muscle lengthens, the leg can gradually be brought inward, closer to midline, so it is aligned with the hip joint.

The client stories that follow will hopefully depict that improving control of the knee's rotation eliminates pain. But you'll notice that the knee wasn't directly treated in any of the cases. Instead, all the answers came from correcting problems at the hip or simply asking the client to stop allowing the knee to collapse in (which means their hip muscles must work better).

The take-home message here is that knee pain is often due to uncontrolled inward rotation of the knee joint. This is usually due to poor control of the femur but can also be the result of poor foot mechanics (see *Fixing You: Foot & Ankle Pain*). The big three hip flexors can contribute to this, especially in the face of weak external rotators of the hip (i.e., the gluteals). All of these muscles originate at the pelvis. Beginning here typically fixes most if not all knee pain.

CLIENT CONNECTION: BYRON'S BAD KNEES

Byron was in his thirties and an avid mountain biker, hiker, and runner. He complained of both knees hurting during all three activities for several months. He would lay off the exercise and the pain would diminish but would return again once he resumed. He had a big competition coming up and wanted to participate but could not complete his training.

His pain primarily happened when riding up steep hills and walking or running more than three miles. The pain was mostly in the front of his knee and sometimes the inner portion.

While assessing Byron's knees, I found his gluteals were weak and the front muscles of his hip were overly tight. Watching his cycling form, I saw his knees collapse in during the downstroke. This is typical riding form for drafting purposes, but it can contribute to knee pain.

Finally, Byron's thigh bones were structurally rotated outward (retroversion). It's important to understand that because his thigh bones were rotated outward, he experienced stress to his knees if those same bones were allowed to rotate in during his sports. That's exactly what was happening.

During cycling, the knees move inward to draft. This put Byron's hips and knees at a biomechanical disadvantage because they were not built to be in this position. Likewise, after approximately three miles of running, Byron's hip muscles would fatigue and allow the knees to begin collapsing inward. The same went for his long hikes.

The Fixing You Approach for Byron's Knees

One of the first things we addressed were Byron's gluteal muscles to control the rotation of his thigh bones during sports (Gluteal Pumps and Side-Lying Clamshells). We also experimented with his seat position, moving it back 1/2 inch to unload the stress to the knees.

Once Byron's gluteal strength improved, we could transfer his new awareness to his sports. I taught him to walk and then run while activating his gluteal muscles (Walk the Walk).

With some further tweaking of his running and cycling style, his knee pain was gone after four visits. Soon he was cycling 40 miles, running 12 miles, and going on 15-mile hikes without pain.

CLIENT CONNECTION: CAROL'S COLLAPSING KNEE

Carol was a 50-something mother who spent most of her day bending and sitting in low chairs at a daycare center. She went on frequent walks with her husband but noticed over the course of two weeks that her right knee began to hurt. The week prior to seeing me, she began to experience shooting pains into her right knee that were almost debilitating.

Our initial evaluation revealed weak gluteals and a thigh bone that rotated in when she walked; the muscles controlling this rotation were tight. Because her day involved a lot of standing and sitting, I decided to watch her sit down. Her right knee instantly collapsed toward her left (Figure 2.25). When she stood up, the right knee pressed against the left while pushing up.

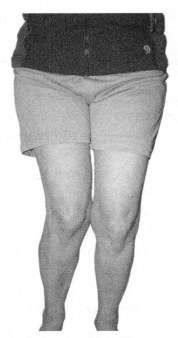 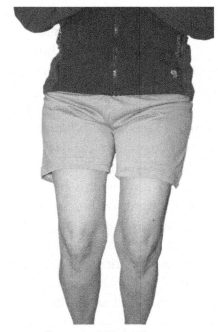

Collapsing Right Knee   **Corrected Right Knee**

Figure 2.25 The image on the left shows poor alignment of the right knee when squatting. This caused pain. Correcting knee alignment to prevent excessive inward rotation eliminated her knee pain.

The Fixing You Approach for Carol's Knee

Because Carol's day involved moving from standing to sitting in low chairs and back up again, I felt this was the activity we needed to focus on first; repeatedly collapsing the knee during the day had taken its toll.

To fix this, I simply told her not to allow the right knee to collapse in when sitting down or standing up. Lo and behold, no knee pain! Repeatedly practicing this would tighten and strengthen key hip muscles that had become either weak or long. This is an important idea to note: Improving movement habits restores individual muscle strength and length. If you think of our chronic pain cycle, then we can reverse the arrows and call it a perpetual healing cycle instead!

The next step was to address everything that was feeding this poor habit, including stretching the muscles on the front of her hip that helped rotate the femur inward (TFL & Quadriceps Stretch). These were extremely tight.

Then I taught her how to strengthen the gluteal muscles to help prevent the internal rotation of her thigh bone (Gluteal Pumps and Side-Lying Clamshells). The gluteals were very weak, and she could only perform three repetitions of the Side-Lying Clamshells exercise before her pelvis began to compensate by rocking backward.

We also addressed her walking habits (Walk the Walk). Carol walked with her hips resting behind her feet and knees. She essentially used her hamstrings to pull her over her feet rather than using her gluteals to propel her forward. Her knees were locked while doing this. All of these habits contributed to her gluteals' underperformance and poor knee function.

To fix this, I asked her to take smaller steps and shift her weight forward when her foot met the ground. When the foot strikes on the ground, the knee should be slightly bent or soft with the hip over the foot. With a little practice, she felt her gluteals turn on at foot strike

Carol slept on her left side, which meant that her right knee would drop down to the left leg during the night, stretching and weakening those same gluteal muscles. I asked Carol to sleep with a pillow between her knees. This prevented the right knee from falling down to the left knee while she was sleeping.

After two treatment sessions, her knee pain was completely gone, her walk had improved, and the muscles in the front of her hips had almost completely stretched out. She could sit and stand without any knee pain, and the right knee did not collapse in. Best of all, she could continue her walks with her husband without pain.

SIMPLIFYING HIP & KNEE PAIN

Hopefully, you're seeing a pattern emerge. One of the biggest problems contributing to knee pain is lack of control of the thigh bone. The muscles in the front of the pelvis typically become tight or dominant, consequently rotating the thigh bone inward. This often happens because of our movement habits. The muscles in the back of the hips become lengthened and/or weak due to a number of reasons, which allows the internal rotation to happen. These muscles are supposed to balance against the front pelvic muscles.

Essentially, the same set of circumstances is behind hip or pelvic pain. Instead of the imbalances affecting the knees, they cause hip pain. Why? My guess is that in different people, one of these joints is more susceptible to excessive movement. Therefore, pain results. This could be due to a variety a reasons, most of which stem from movement habits created over the years. Restoring balance to the muscles on the front and back of the pelvis eliminates hip and knee pain.

You'll notice that I mentioned many muscles and other possibilities for poor joint function at the roots of hip or knee pain, yet the only tests I've given you are to determine whether your gluteal muscles are working and whether you have a rotated pelvis. To test every possible muscle and joint issue would be beyond the scope of this book. That's for professionals. My point is to help you realize that if you've found either of these issues occurring, there's a good chance they are a large part of the problems creating your pain. Together with walking, standing, or sitting habits, these issues are central to solving hip or knee pain. The exercises in Section 3 will correct these problems for you.

So, now we've covered just about everything you need to know to fix your hip and knee pain. I know it sounds a little daunting, but if you remember that most hip and knee pain is caused by tightness of the big three hip flexors rotating the pelvis forward or the knees inward and weak muscles in the back of the pelvis allowing this to happen, you'll get where you need to go.

Also please remember that even though performing the exercises in Section 3 will reduce or eliminate your pain, it will always come back if you do not also fix your movement habits. These typically involve asymmetrical weight-bearing or poor walking mechanics. Once you can fix these issues, your pain will evaporate permanently.

HELPFUL DAILY TIPS

Fixing hip and knee pain requires diligence about correcting bad habits during the day and night. Here are some helpful tips that have benefited my clients.

During the Day

I cannot emphasize enough the importance of mastering gluteal muscle activation while walking and standing throughout the day. The easiest way to remember this is to stand symmetrically with your knees soft rather than locked into extension. While walking, remember to keep the hip and trunk over the foot and knee slightly bent at foot strike. This often involves taking shorter steps.

In the case of knee pain, the key is to not allow the knees to collapse inward while walking, sitting, kneeling, going up and down stairs, etc. Also, try to point the toes outward slightly when walking, standing, or sitting to see if this decreases your knee pain. If it does, then an ante- or retroverted femur may be contributing to your problem.

It's difficult to remember to do this often enough due to the distractions of work and life pulling at you every minute. For this reason, I recommend creating reminders such as stickers on your watch, phone, dashboard of your car—anything you look at frequently to remind you to walk correctly to engage the gluteal muscles. You could also wear your watch on your opposite wrist, or set up a timer on your phone or computer, or wear a special ring or bracelet to help you remember to fix your bad habits contributing to pain.

Sitting

Periodically check how you are bearing weight while sitting in your chair. Is one cheek loaded more than another? Is one leg rotated inward? Does one hip seem to be more hiked up than the other? When bending down to sit, are one or both knees collapsing in? How about when standing up: do your knees briefly drift in together? If so, begin fixing these problems.

Exercising

While running, working on an elliptical machine, cycling, or rowing, notice whether one or both knees tend to collapse inward and correct it. It may be time to slow down or reduce resistance to fix the mechanics of your movement. Once corrected, you can gradually increase weight or speed again as long as you continue with good form.

> When exercising on machines, **watch, listen,** and **feel** whether your form is symmetrical.

Another common problem is weight-bearing excessively through one leg or shifting your body over one foot more than the other. I often exercise without music so I can hear the difference between how my left and right foot are hitting the ground when running. Perhaps having someone check your form for symmetry would be helpful.

Sleeping

An easy fix for knee or hip pain is to place a pillow between the knees and feet if you sleep on your side. This reduces internal rotation at both the hip and knee, which relieves stress to the tissues involved. When the knee is allowed to drop down, the external rotator muscles of the hip that act on the thigh bone are lengthened and consequently put at a mechanical disadvantage to heal. Placing a pillow between the knees also reduces rotational torque at the knee joint, which permits healing to occur. This is especially helpful for those with wide hips.

CONCLUSION

Hip and knee pain is ubiquitous in our society. I believe much of this stems from habits such as locking our knees to conserve strength or asymmetrically standing or running, which creates a rotated pelvis. Our muscles eventually adapt to these movement patterns, creating abnormal wear and tear on our joints.

You've learned about some major muscle groups in the front and back of the pelvis and how they should balance each other to maintain optimal biomechanics of the hip joint and leg bone. Most cases I see involve weak gluteals in the presence of tight muscles in the front of the pelvis. This contributes to excessive internal rotation of the leg bone or the femoral head sliding forward in the socket, which causes hip or groin pain. SI joint pain can also happen as a result of this because the pelvic bones can actually become torqued from these asymmetrical forces.

Something you should also keep in mind is the fact that many people's femurs are structurally rotated inward (anteversion) or outward (retroversion), which further complicates hip and knee mechanics. This can't be changed; however, knowledge of this rotation can help you avoid injury and optimize performance by working within the boundaries of your physical limitations and learning to use them to your advantage.

Regarding knee pain, by far the most common problem I see involves the femur internally rotating too much. Again this relates to the hip muscles' function because many muscles controlling rotation of the knee joint are found at the hip.

Correcting these issues will require you to pay attention to how you're standing, sitting, walking, or running. Once you can see what's wrong, it becomes easier to fix it. Fixing your habits will be a large part of eliminating your pain. Initially, you'll feel awkward changing how you walk or stand. At the same time, however, your pain should decrease. This should tell you that your "natural" habits are actually hurting you and must be replaced with seemingly "unnatural," but correct, movements to fix your pain. This, together with the corrective exercises in Section 3, should completely eliminate your pain and get you back to doing the things you love!

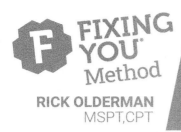

RICK OLDERMAN
MSPT,CPT

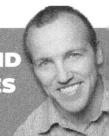

FIXING CHRONIC AND
RECURRING INJURIES
SINCE 1996

**You have been granted FREE ACCESS
to the exercise videos for this book!**

**Learn how to perform the exercise correctly!
Get faster results! Feel better sooner!**

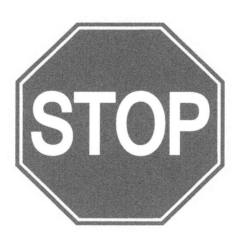

Visit www.FixingYouBooks.com/hipkneepain

Enter the code: **gluteals**

3 | CORRECTIVE EXERCISES

I've been a few places like that where I've thought, "A BREAKTHROUGH is possible here. This is the place for the EXERCISES that will bring me to WHERE I WANT TO BE."

—JOSEPH CAMPBELL

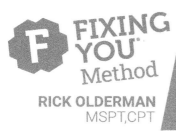
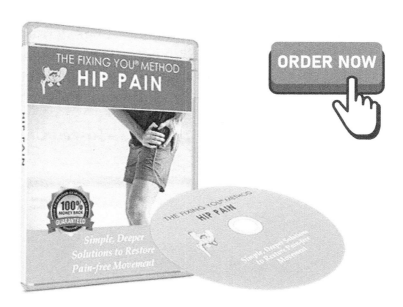

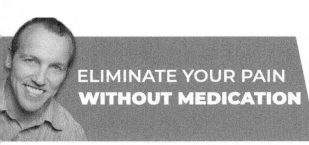 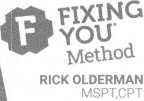
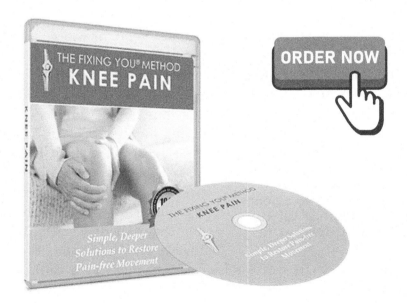

The following exercises are meant to develop strength and improve range of motion. If you find a particular exercise difficult, chances are it's because of weakness or movement dysfunction. Take that as a cue that you need help here and therefore should practice it until you've mastered it. Good form is critical.

If you find an exercise that feels good, then do it as often as you can. Trust your body, it knows what it likes! In particular, the stretches should always feel good. During the first week or two, I typically begin with stretches such as All-Fours Rocking Stretch or TFL & Quadriceps Stretch. Restoring range of motion and getting things moving the way they should always helps healing and reduces pain. The other reason to begin with stretching is that it will allow you to identify the exercise(s) that are doing the most good for you.

> **Resist the temptation** to push too far too fast, and remember to **listen to your body**. If you feel pain, stop!

Stretching exercises are generally held for 30–60 seconds. Performing 2–5 repetitions is usually all that's needed to experience a positive effect. I typically ask my clients to commit to performing their stretches as often as possible (2–5 times each day) during the first week or two to aggressively reduce their symptoms. In fact, because the TFL & Quadriceps Stretch is so effective, I ask my clients to perform this every time they experience pain. It should always feel good to perform the stretching exercises, so this really shouldn't be a hard sell. You should feel that your pain has decreased as a result. After the symptoms have abated, you can cut down on the frequency of the exercises and find the ideal number of times needed to keep your body corrected. I recommend doing them at least first thing in the morning and last thing before bed.

> **Poor form or posture** during strength training can promote pain. Understand your poor habits and **counter them with good form.**

After the stretching phase, begin strengthening. Add one exercise at a time to focus both on getting it right and to test whether your pain is made worse by it. Most likely, you'll begin with the Gluteal Pumps. If your pain is made worse, then either your technique is incorrect or it's not the right exercise for you. Pay attention to how you are performing the exercise. Read the instructions carefully and watch the video clips on the Fixing You website. Once you are successfully performing the exercise, then layer on the next. Each time you add a new strengthening exercise, do not change anything else about your program in order to isolate that which may be causing pain.

> **If you are weight training,** you may find that you must **temporarily decrease the weight** you are using. It's okay—fixing your hip and/or knee is the **bigger picture.**

Strengthening exercises generally require 5–10 repetitions for 1–2 sets or until fatigue or compensatory movements occur. Just a little bit of strengthening is needed to effect a positive change. As always, quality is more important than quantity. Strengthening exercises only need to be performed 2–3 times a day during the initial 1–2 week period. After that you can devote less time, since you will have identified and corrected movement habits that were contributing to your pain.

Any exercises that cause or increase pain are either incorrect for your problem or are being performed incorrectly. Videos of all exercises can be viewed on **www.FixingYou.net** by typing in the code found in the back of this book.

The following exercises will address most hip and knee problems and offer quick relief. Begin with those focusing on stretching or range of motion and then progress to strengthening exercises once you have mastered them.

One last word of advice, however. These exercises will only be part of your solution. You must pay attention to, and correct, your pain-producing habits. You cannot permanently fix your pain otherwise.

TOP 5 HIP & KNEE CORRECTION EXERCISES

1 **TFL & Quadriceps Stretch** reduces pelvic rotation.

2 **Side-Lying Clamshells** improve hip muscle strength.

3 **All-Fours Rocking Stretch** passively restores normal hip mechanics.

4 **Gluteal Pumps** restore proper gluteal strength.

5 **Walk the Walk** activates proper gluteal function and improves femur tracking while walking.

TFL & QUADRICEPS STRETCH

This exercise stretches the muscles that attach to the front of the pelvis and affect pelvic, thigh, and therefore knee rotation. It also develops lower abdominal strength and therefore control of pelvic rotation. I highly encourage you to watch the video clip of this exercise on the Fixing You website to understand precisely how it should be done. In Level 1, the goal is to allow one leg to lie flat on the table without the spine arching off the table. This focuses on one of the big three hip flexors. In Level 2, the thigh should be able to lie flat on the table with knee bent to 90–100 degrees, with back flat, and without the pelvis rotating forward. Often I add a 1- to 3-pound ankle weight to the lowered leg to increase the stretch to the muscles. This is done only after the client has shown they can stabilize their pelvis and spine correctly, though.

> If you have back pain, please read **Fixing You: Back Pain** for specific instructions about the root causes of your pain.

THE FIXING YOU METHOD—LEVEL 1

Lie on your back with both knees drawn to your chest. Hold the left knee with your left hand and arm. Place your right hand on the bony prominence (ASIS) of your right hip (see video clip for further instruction). With knee bent, slowly lower your right foot to the table. Next, slide your right foot away from your hips, straightening the knee. Stop if your spine arches off the table or your pelvis rotates up from the table into your right hand. See if you can keep your back flat and your pelvis from rotating while your right leg rests straight on the table. Pull your left knee into your chest with more force if necessary to help you keep your lower back flat. Visualize the hip-flexor muscles lengthening away from the ASIS of the pelvis. Note whether you feel a gentle stretch in the upper thigh close to the hip bone. Hold the stretch for 30–60 seconds and switch legs. Sometimes placing a 5- to 10-pound weight on your right thigh close to your knee will add to the stretch. Do this only if your spine is not arching and your pelvis is stable and not rotated forward. If you have difficulty performing this exercise, remain at this level until your abdominal strength is able to stabilize your pelvis and back adequately or until you can easily keep your leg straight on the table with your lower spine flat and do not feel a stretch in the front of your thigh on either leg. At this point, you can move to Level 2.

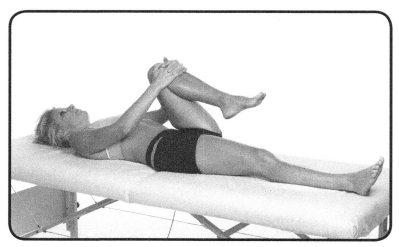

TFL & Quadriceps Stretch—Level 1, end position

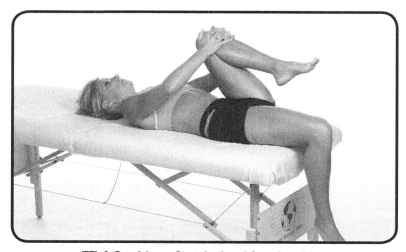

TFL & Quadriceps Stretch—Level 2, end position

THE FIXING YOU METHOD—LEVEL 2

Begin as you did in Level 1 and slowly lower your right leg; keep your knee bent at 90 degrees as your leg lowers off the edge of the table while monitoring the ASIS with your fingers. Stop if you feel your hip bone begin to rotate forward or your lower back begins to arch off the table. Contract your abdominal muscles or pull the opposite knee harder into your chest to prevent your pelvis from rolling forward as you lower your leg down. Feel for a stretch at the base of the hip bone you're monitoring and/or in the upper thigh. Feel your leg gradually lower as your muscles lengthen against your stabilized pelvis. Do not push your leg down; instead, allow gravity to slowly pull it down. Exhale forcefully to assist your lower abdominals in stabilizing your lumbar spine and pelvis. Stop if you cannot stabilize the lumbar spine against the lowering leg.

Note: If your foot rotates out as you lower your leg, your ITB is probably tight. Simply rotate the foot so it faces forward in order to stretch the ITB.

Also, if you're having trouble maintaining the stretch while keeping your lumbar spine flat on the table, lightly rest the lowered foot on a stool or other object at the point where you can feel the stretch in the front of your leg and your back stays flat.

COMMON ERRORS

• If you experience back pain when stretching, your abdominals are not adequately stabilizing your spine and your pelvis is rotating more than it should (see *Fixing You: Back Pain*). Try pulling the opposite knee up further to your chest to assist with rotating the pelvis back into the table.

• Knee pain may result in the leg that you're lowering if the stretch is too aggressive. Either prevent your leg from lowering to the point of knee pain or slide your leg out to the side and then lower it. Find a position where you can experience a pain-free stretch. Your goal will then be to gradually work your way back in toward your trunk so you can lower the leg straight down instead of out to the side.

SIDE-LYING CLAMSHELLS

This exercise restores strength to the back portion of the gluteus medius. This helps with knee tracking and counters the pull of the TFL. This is not a big range-of-motion exercise. Keep it relatively small. Those with retroverted femurs (usually men) will generally be able to work in a higher leg position than those with anteverted femurs (usually women). Regardless, only raise your leg to the point where your pelvis doesn't rock backward and you feel a good contraction in the muscles in the back of your hip.

THE FIXING YOU METHOD

Lie on your right side with knees bent and spine in a neutral position. Draw your belly button in toward your spine to engage your lower abdominals to stabilize your spine and pelvis. Be sure your hip bones are stacked on top of each other. Put your left fingers on the back of your left hip to monitor the contraction of your muscles. Keeping your heels touching, raise your left knee while pivoting on the left heel, creating an arc with the left knee. Do not allow the hips to roll back; keep them stacked. This is very important, so continually monitor them. Feel the muscles turn on under your right fingers. Lower your knee only until the point the muscles turn off—usually only 1/4–1/2 inch—then use the muscles in the back of your hip to raise your knee back up. We want these muscles to stay turned on as long as possible. Maintain the contraction while you continue to rotate your knee up and down in a small range of motion. Stop if back or hip pain occurs or you are unable to maintain good form. Perform 3–15 repetitions or until you become fatigued or compensations occur, such as the pelvis rocking backward. Switch sides.

COMMON ERRORS

•   If your top hip rocks back in order to get your knee up in air, make the movement smaller so your hip does not rock backward.

•   If back or hip pain occurs, make sure the top heel is resting on the bottom heel. Try placing a towel or pillow between your knees. Limit the range of motion to a smaller range. Check to confirm your hips are stacked on top of each other. See *Fixing You: Back Pain.*

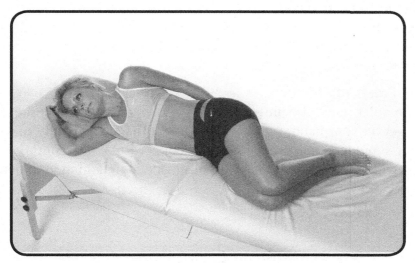

Side-Lying Clamshells, start position

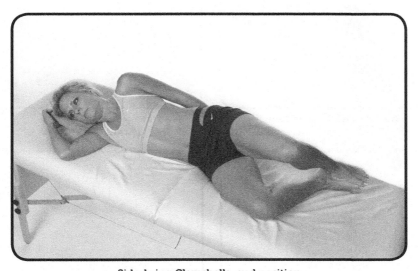

Side-Lying Clamshells, end position

ALL-FOURS ROCKING STRETCH

This exercise passively restores normal hip mechanics and feels great for the hips when performed properly. Move only in a pain-free range of motion. People with ankle problems can perform this stretch so their feet hang off the edge of a bed.

THE FIXING YOU METHOD

With a flat (neutral) spine and pelvis and your belly button drawn in, get on your hands and knees with your hands generally under your shoulders and knees under your hips. Rock back onto your feet while keeping your hands in place and maintaining your neu-

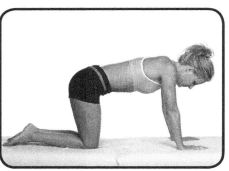

All-Fours Rocking Stretch,
start position

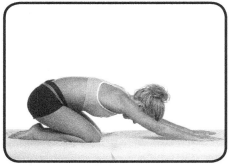

All-Fours Rocking Stretch,
end position

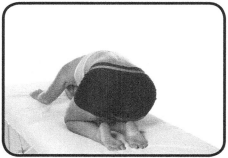

Alternative All-Fours Rocking Stretch,
rotated pelvis error

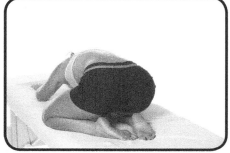

Alternative All-Fours Rocking Stretch,
rotated pelvis correction

tral spine. Hold for 5 breaths. Repeat 5–10 times.

Note any stretching in the muscles in the back of your hip or pelvis or front of your quadriceps.

MODIFICATION FOR PELVIC ROTATION PROBLEMS

If your pelvis is rotated, you'll find that one hip doesn't rock back as far as the other side. For instance, your left hip may not come down to the heel as far as your right hip (as shown in the photos on the opposite page). In this case, keep your foot in position but scoot your left knee out to the side about 2–3 inches. Rock back and feel with your hands that the hip depth is more symmetrical. Find the right distance to scoot out your knee until you feel both hips are symmetrical. Repeat 5–10 times, then scoot your left knee back in where you began; recheck your hips by reaching back to feel the distance from the hip to the heel. Continue to repeat this sequence until you feel your pelvis is symmetrical. It's often helpful to have someone watch you perform this exercise to assess alignment.

COMMON ERRORS

•   If you feel hip pain while rocking back, then only go to the point just before pain and stop. Repeat this a few times and see whether you are able to go further after the hip has loosened up. If you can get to the bottom but feel pain, again stop short of that pain and work there until there is no pain. Keep retesting to see if you are improving.

•   Make sure you start in the right position. Your knees should be under your hips with the knees separated to allow your stomach to drop between the knees.

•   Always be sure your spine is stabilized by drawing in your belly button.

•   If you have a rotated pelvis, don't forget to scoot the knee out to compensate for the rotated pelvis. It will most likely be on the same side as the hip that can't lower as far as the other side.

GLUTEAL PUMPS

This exercise restores strength to the gluteus maximus. Gluteal strength is critical for proper hip and knee mechanics.

THE FIXING YOU METHOD—LEVEL 1

It's best for everyone to begin at this level because you can more easily isolate the gluteal muscles without compensating through other parts of the body. Lie on your stomach. Bend your right knee to 90 degrees while stabilizing the lumbar spine by drawing in the belly button; if you can't do this, then try Windshield Wip-

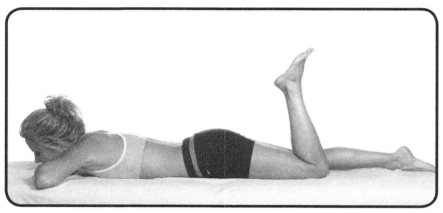

Gluteal Pumps—Level 1, start position

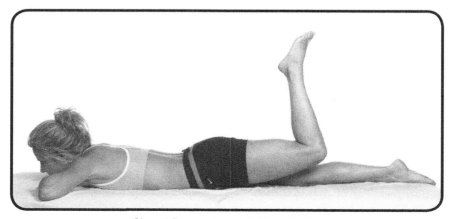

Gluteal Pumps—Level 1, end position

ers—Level 1. Now lift your right leg with the knee bent, focusing on squeezing the gluteus muscles to lift your leg rather than pulling it up with the hamstring muscles or arching the spine. Hold for 2 breaths, then slowly lower your leg with the gluteals in control. Repeat 5–10 repetitions or until fatigued. If this is difficult, try squeezing both gluteal cheeks together then lifting your leg.

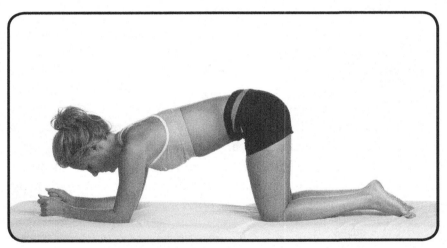

Gluteal Pumps—Level 2, start position

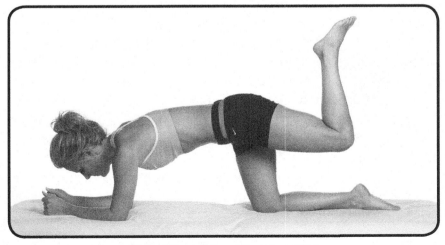

Gluteal Pumps—Level 2, end position

THE FIXING YOU METHOD—LEVEL 2

You can practice Level 2 once you've achieved 10 repetitions of Level 1 without compensating through the spine or using the hamstrings to lift your leg. Assume a position on your elbows and knees with your spine in a flattened (neutral) position. Hold your spine in place by drawing your belly button in toward your spine. Squeeze your gluteals to raise one leg up in the air with knee bent at 90 degrees. Stop at the point where you feel the maximal contraction of these muscles. Your thigh should roughly be in line with your trunk at this point. Slowly lower your leg until you feel the gluteals are not contracting any longer; this will be the lowest point of the range of motion you will work in. Usually this is a small range of motion initially, say, 1/4–1/2 inch. Pump your leg up and down in a small, controlled motion while maintaining the gluteal contraction. Do not lower your leg to the point the gluteals turn off. Make the gluteals fatigue. Perform 10–30 repetitions until fatigue, failure, or compensations occur (such as the spine arching or the hamstrings becoming fatigued instead of the gluteals). Switch sides.

COMMON ERRORS

• You may find your back arches in order to bring your leg up higher. If this happens, stabilize your spine by drawing your belly button in, or don't raise the leg up quite so high.

• If your hamstrings cramp or fatigue, you're lifting using your hamstrings instead of your gluteals. Focus on pulling your leg up by squeezing your rear-end muscles. Keep your hamstrings relatively relaxed. Stretch the front of your thigh muscles so your hamstrings aren't working so hard to bend the knee. Perform the TFL & Quadriceps Stretch or Windshield Wipers—Level 1 to stretch the thigh muscles.

• If back pain occurs after making the appropriate corrections, then please read *Fixing You: Back Pain*.

WALK THE WALK

This exercise improves gluteus maximus function while walking or running. This is important for improving hip and knee mechanics. This is perhaps one of the most important and difficult items to correct. Take your time.

The Fixing You Method

While standing, put your right leg back with your hand on your right gluteal muscles. Contract your gluteal muscles and feel the contraction with your right hand. The contraction you feel is what you will be striving for when walking. Relax the contraction of the right gluteus muscles; step forward with your right foot while unlocking your right knee prior to striking the foot down onto the floor. When your foot strikes, make sure your hips are over

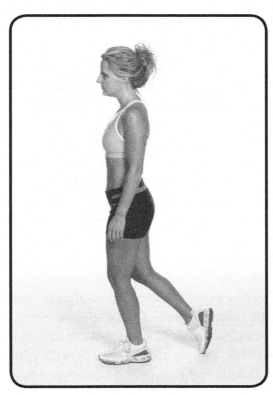

Walk the Walk

your foot, not behind it. It is very likely you will need to take a much shorter step to achieve this. That's okay. When your trunk is over your foot and the knee unlocked at foot strike, you should feel your gluteals turn on. The gluteals should turn on as a consequence of stepping correctly, not because you're making them contract. If you don't feel them turn on, there are three possible causes:

1) Your hip is still too far behind your knee.

2) Your knee is not unlocked.

3) You are not weight-bearing through your arch.

Lean your hips forward over the knee to engage the gluteus muscles. Some of you may need to lift up your back (left) leg to make sure the right hip is over the right foot. Now do you feel it? If not, then bend your knee while bouncing gently or slightly flexing forward at the hip until you can feel the gluteus muscles activate.

One other idea that works well with stubborn gluteals is to stand on one leg with your knee slightly bent and perform a small, single-leg squat to turn on the gluteal muscles. You need only squat about 1/2–1 inch to turn on the gluteal muscles. This almost always gets them to turn on. Once you feel the contraction, move to the other leg. Continue walking, moving into a single-leg mini-squat if necessary until you are able to turn on the gluteals more naturally. Again, the gluteal muscles should activate as a consequence of walking correctly, not because you are squeezing them consciously.

Continue practicing by taking one step—feeling the gluteals engage—then take another step doing the same on the other side. Do not take another step until the gluteals are contracting well. Gradually you will be able to know the gluteals are firing without using your hands. After you feel confident the gluteal muscles are turning on at footstrike, begin standing up straighter and straightening your knee a little more to more closely approximate your old walking style. You should be able to walk looking almost exactly as you did before with only a minor difference but with your gluteal muscles turned on. Practice whenever and wherever you can.

WINDSHIELD WIPERS

This exercise is great for restoring normal range of motion and motor control to the hip joint and muscles. It also develops lower abdominal strength to stabilize the pelvis during leg movements. It will loosen and stretch the TFL and rectus femoris as well. Ideally, your legs should rotate about 30–45 degrees in both directions, unless you have retroverted or anteverted femurs.

THE FIXING YOU METHOD—PART 1

Lie on your stomach with hands under your ASISs to monitor movement. Use a pillow under your hips if you have back pain in this position. Be sure your hips are level and equal pressure is in both hands. Bend your knee to 90 degrees so your foot is approximately above the knee. Stop if you feel your hip bone pressure on your hands change, your lower spine arches, or you feel pain in your lower back. If these compensations are occurring, then your muscles are tighter than your spine's ability to stabilize against their tension. Do not bend your knee further if you encounter any of these problems. Instead, lower your foot back down and draw your belly button in toward your spine or exhale briskly to activate your abdominal muscles while slowly bending your knee again. Stop at the point where any compensations occur. See if

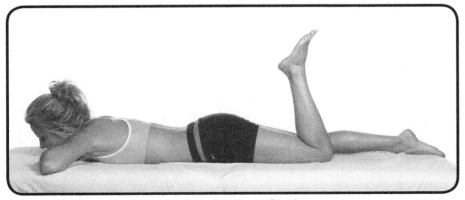

Windshield Wipers, Part 1

you can move past the barrier without compromising your form. Your first goal will be to bend your knee 90–110 degrees without any compensations occurring in your pelvis or spine. Repeat on the other leg. Once you are successful you can move on to Part 2 of this exercise. Depending on how tight your leg muscles are, this may take some time.

THE FIXING YOU METHOD—PART 2

Lie on your stomach with hands under your ASISs to monitor movement. Be sure your hips are level and equal pressure is in

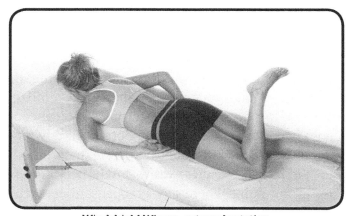

Windshield Wipers, external rotation

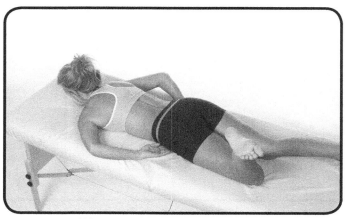

Windshield Wipers, internal rotation

both hands. Use a pillow under your hips if you experience back pain in this position (see *Fixing You: Back Pain*). Bend your right knee to approximately 90 degrees of flexion. Now slowly rotate your right foot and lower leg away from center. Stop if your right hip bone pushes down into your hand or raises off your left hand. Return and slowly move your right foot inward to the other direction—creating a slow, windshield-wiper motion with your lower leg. Again, stop if the right or left hip bone pressure on your hands change. At the points where the pelvis moves, contract your lower abdominals to stabilize your pelvis and/or exhale briskly to activate them. See if you can go further now that it is stabilized. Rotating the foot across midline (external rotation) will help stretch the TFL. Repeat for 5–10 repetitions and then perform on the other leg.

COMMON ERRORS

•   If you experience back or hip pain when your foot is raised, the muscles in front of your thighs may be tight. Go back to Part 1 and correct your hip and back compensations while bending your knee. You can also place a pillow or two under your waist and try again, but ultimately, we want this exercise to be performed without pillows under your waist. Also, you may not be able to stabilize your pelvis well enough with your lower abdominals. Draw your belly button in toward your spine to better stabilize your pelvis. Stop if you experience pain or pelvic movement. Do not move on to Part 2 until you can perform Part 1 without pain.

•   If you experience back or hip pain when moving your foot side to side, your pelvis is probably moving too much. Stabilize better or decrease the range of motion until it is pain free and/or stabilized.

•   If your hamstrings cramp, they're working too hard against tight muscles in the front of the thighs. Try a pillow under your stomach or stretch the muscles in front of the leg using the TFL & Quadriceps Stretch.

HIP TUBES

This exercise also strengthens the gluteal muscles and translates strength gains to walking or sports because performing it correctly requires stabilization of the entire body in a standing position. It is an advanced-level exercise and should only be performed after mastering Side-Lying Clamshells.

The Fixing You Method

If you have difficulty balancing, begin this exercise without an exercise tube and lightly hold on to a stable surface for assistance. Stand and place an exercise tube or stretch band under both feet where your heels meet the arches of your feet. Raise the handles by bending your elbows as in the picture. Raise your right foot off the floor approximately 1/2 inch. Slightly rotate your right knee outward while maintaining a square (neutral) pelvis and facing forward. Soften the left knee and be sure you are bearing weight through the arch of your left foot. While keeping your right foot lifted 1/2 inch from the floor, move it out to the side and then back in (4–12 inches). Make the movement smooth and slow while maintaining your square pelvis, soft left knee, and bearing your weight through the left arch; maintain a tall spine without leaning. Perform 15 repetitions without allowing the right foot to touch the floor. Switch legs. Repeat 3 times on each leg.

Common Errors

•   Hip or knee pain can result if your pelvis is permitted to rotate while pumping the moving leg. Maintain a neutral, forward-facing position.

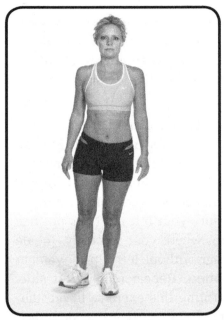

Hip Strengthening, start position

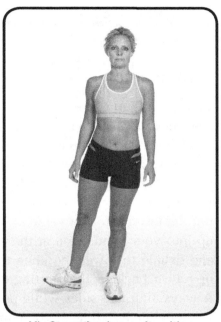

Hip Strengthening, end position

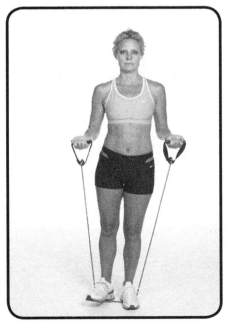

Hip Tubes, start position

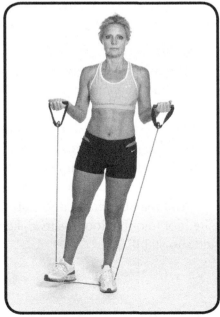

Hip Tubes, end position

KNEE WOBBLES

This exercise strengthens the lower abdominals' ability to stabilize against pelvic rotation. The knees should be able to rotate out about 30–40 degrees without pelvic movement.

THE FIXING YOU METHOD

Lie on your back with knees bent, flattened lumbar spine, and hands on your hip bones (ASISs) to monitor movement. Engage your lower abdominals by drawing your belly button in toward your spine and/or exhaling by pushing the belly button toward your spine. Slowly lower your right knee out to the side, monitoring the left hip for movement. Be sure your left hip does not rise up into your hand. Stop at the point where your hip rises. Inhale and exhale to lower the knee further without left hip movement or return back to the starting position. Repeat on the left side. Always alternate sides while performing this exercise to reestablish a pelvic baseline. If you continually work the same side, then the opposite hip will gradually rise and you won't know it. If you notice that one hip stays down more easily than the other, it could mean you have a rotated pelvis.

COMMON ERRORS

• If one hip rises too soon, stabilize using your lower abdominals. Under no circumstances allow the hip to come up as this just reinforces the pelvic rotation.

• You may feel the opposite hip stay down, but when you return to the starting position, you feel that opposite hip lower back toward the floor. This means the hip is creeping up without your awareness. Develop your sensitivity to discern this movement.

• You may be tempted to stabilize the pelvis by pressing the opposite foot into the floor. Instead, keep the leg relaxed; use your abdominals to stabilize.

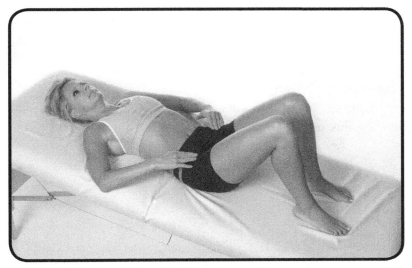

Knee Wobbles, start position

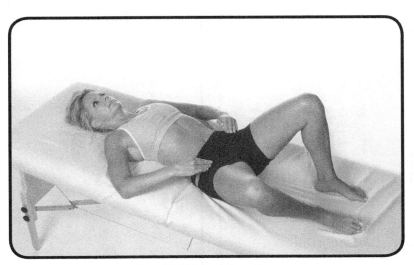

Knee Wobbles, end position

SINGLE-LEG STANDING

This exercise strengthens core muscles and prevents poor habits associated with pelvic and leg movements during walking. This exercise is best performed in front of a mirror or with someone watching you from behind to assess your form—preferably a physical therapist.

THE FIXING YOU METHOD

While standing, bring one knee forward and up to approximately 70–90 degrees of hip flexion. Be sure your pelvis or your stance

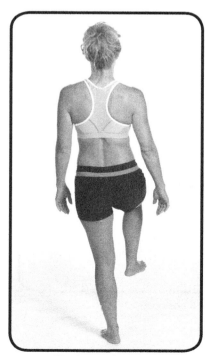 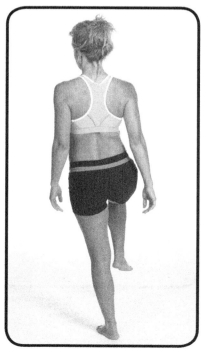

Single-Leg Standing   Single-Leg Standing, error

knee doesn't excessively rotate by drawing your belly button in toward your spine to stabilize it. Feel your hip muscles (gluteals) and thigh muscles stabilize your stance leg. Breathe for 2–3 breaths and then slowly lower your leg back down without allowing your pelvis to rotate. Draw your belly button toward your spine to stabilize your pelvis and leg while alternating legs—like a slow march. Stop whenever you feel pain and note how high your leg can go before feeling pain in order to assess your progress.

COMMON ERRORS

• Try to not allow the pelvis or stance leg to rotate while lifting the leg as this reinforces excessive pelvic or spine rotation when walking. Be precise and take it very slow to analyze yourself.

• Be sure to engage the gluteals on the stance leg to help stabilize the hip.

ITB STRETCH

This exercise helps stretch the ITB and possibly the TFL and rectus femoris muscles if they're tight too. The ITB can also be stretched performing the TFL & Quadriceps Stretch.

THE FIXING YOU METHOD

Lie on your stomach with both legs extended and knees, heels, and toes together. Slowly bend both legs keeping the knees, heels, and toes together. Do not allow the toes of one foot to rotate away from the other foot. Also do not allow your legs to drift to one side as you bend your knees; keep them centered. Bend your knees to 90–110 degrees, feeling for a stretch in the outer portion of the thigh or knee. Be sure your pelvis and lumbar spine remain stabilized and there is no back strain. Maintain the stretch for 30–60 seconds, then slowly lower your legs. Repeat 3–5 times.

COMMON ERRORS

• Both legs may veer to the right or left when performing this exercise. Have a friend critique your form to be sure you are symmetrically bending your knees, heels, and toes together.

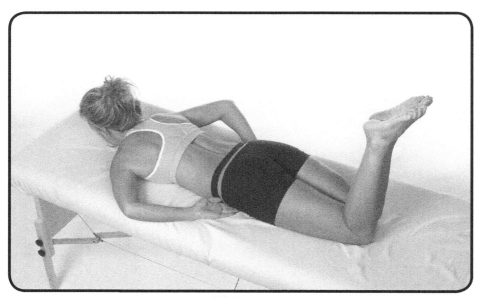

ITB Stretch

FIXING YOU: HIP & KNEE PAIN

GLOSSARY

abdominal muscles
Trunk muscles that help to rotate and flex the spine. The abdominal muscles are composed of:

rectus abdominus: Originates at the pelvis and inserts into the sternum as well as ribs 5–7. This muscle flexes the spine or assists in posteriorly tilting the pelvis.

external obliques: One of the abdominal muscles responsible for rotation and flexion of the spine. Developing external oblique strength is important for spinal stabilization against movement faults.

internal obliques: One of the abdominal muscles responsible for rotation and flexion of the spine. Developing internal oblique strength is important for spinal stabilization against movement faults.

transversus abdominus: An important spinal-stabilizing muscle.

abducting
Moving away from the midline of the body out to the side. For instance, when moving a leg out to the side, the leg is abducting.

abduction
A position that results from abducting an appendage. For example, a leg held out to the side is said to be in abduction.

adducting
Moving toward the body. For example, the process of bringing the leg back to the side of the body from abduction is said to be adducting the leg. An easy way to remember this is adducting adds to the body.

adduction
The position of an appendage closer to the body relative to abduction.

anterior
In front of or forward; the opposite of posterior. For instance, an anterior pelvic tilt occurs when the top of the pelvis is tilted forward.

anterior cruciate ligament (ACL)
This ligament in the center of the knee runs from the femur to the

tibia. Some fibers also blend into the meniscus.

anterior knee pain syndrome (AKPS)—See patellofemoral pain syndrome.

anterior pelvic tilt
Occurs when the top of the pelvis is anteriorly rotated. The effect of the anterior tilt increases spinal extension.

anteversion (femoral)
A structural internal twisting of the femur that points the knees inward when the femur is correctly aligned in the hip socket.

ASIS (anterior superior iliac spine)—See pelvis.

extending
The act of straightening a joint or reversing a flexed position. Extending a knee involves straightening the knee joint.

extension
Describes a straight joint position relative to a flexed position.

external obliques—See abdominal muscles.

external rotation
Rotating the anterior surface of a bone or joint away from the midline of the body; also referred to as lateral rotation. Externally rotating the leg involves turning the leg away from the body so the knee or foot faces outward.

femoral anteversion—See anteversion.

femoral head—See femur.

femoral retroversion—See retroversion.

femur
The thigh bone. This bone has a head (femoral head) that inserts into the hip to form the hip joint. The distal end joins with the tibia and patella to form the knee joint.

fibula
One of the two bones of the lower leg. The outer distal portion forms the lateral bone of the ankle.

flexion
Describes a position that is flexed relative to neutral or extension. A knee is in flexion when it is bent.

foot-strike pattern
How the foot interacts with the ground when walking.

gluteals
A collective term for the gluteus maximus and gluteus medius.

> **gluteus maximus:** This hip muscle runs from the pelvis and inserts into the ITB and femur at the hip joint. Its actions include leg extension, external rotation, and guiding the femoral head in the hip socket.

> **gluteus medius:** This hip muscle originates around the border of the anterior through posterior portions of the pelvis and inserts onto the femur. The anterior fibers medially rotate the leg, the posterior fibers laterally rotate the leg, and all work together to abduct the leg.

hamstrings
Muscles on the back of the leg that flex the knee. When the gluteus maximus is weak and poorly controlling hip extension, the hamstrings may help with this motion.

> **semitendinosus:** This hamstring muscle originates at the pelvis and inserts on the medial surface of the body of the tibia. It flexes and medially rotates the knee and can assist with medial rotation of the hip.

> **semimembranosus:** This hamstring muscle originates at the pelvis and inserts on the medial surface of the tibia. It flexes and medially rotates the knee and can assist with medial rotation of the hip.

> **biceps femoris:** Lateral hamstring muscles composed of:

>> **short head:** Originates along the femur and inserts with the long head onto the lateral side of the fibula and lateral portion of the tibia.

>> **long head:** Originates at the pelvis and blends with the short head to its insertion on the lower leg.

hip
The joint where the femur and pelvis meet. This is a ball-and-socket joint, similar to the shoulder, that can move in many directions.

hyperextension
A joint that extends too far or too easily is said to be hyperextended.

hypermobile joint
A joint that has too much motion, which may or may not be well controlled, is said to be hypermobile. A hypermobile joint often occurs near a hypomobile joint.

hypomobile joint
A joint that has too little motion. When a joint does not move well, other joints above or below it typically must compensate by becoming hypermobile in order to achieve functional movement.

iliotibial band (ITB)
A dense band of noncontractile tissue, called fascia, that covers the gluteal region and into which the tensor fascia lata and gluteus maximus are attached. Distally the ITB inserts into the kneecap, tibia and fibular head.

ITB-friction syndrome
Irritation of the ITB that can cause hip or knee pain.

iliac crest—See pelvis.

ilium—See pelvis.

impinged
Pinched or compressed, usually between two bones. For instance, a nerve may become impinged if it is pinched between two vertebrae.

internal obliques—See abdominal muscles.

internal rotation
Rotating the anterior surface of a bone or joint toward the midline of the body; also referred to as medial rotation. Internally rotating the leg involves turning the leg in toward the body so the knee or foot faces inward.

ischial tuberosity pain syndrome
Characterized by chronic irritation of the origin of the hamstrings at the ischial tuberosity.

joint capsule
A dense, fibrous connective tissue that surrounds our joints, providing stability and assisting with coordinating movement.

labrum
A ring of thick cartilage around the hip sockets that deepens the socket and provides stability for the femoral heads as they move in the sockets.

ligament
A fibrous, noncontractile tissue that connects bone to bone. Ligaments help stabilize joints.

movement dysfunction
A way of moving that can cause pain. For instance, when sitting down and allowing one or both knees to collapse inward, this movement dysfunction will cause knee pain.

movement fault—See movement dysfunction.

osteoarthritis
Involves joint degradation of the surface or underlying bone.

patella
The kneecap.

patellofemoral syndrome (anterior knee pain syndrome)
The name given to a cluster of anterior knee pain symptoms that are exacerbated with prolonged sitting or climbing stairs.

pelvis
A term given to a collection of bones on which our spine rests and with which our legs articulate. It is composed of:

> **sacrum:** A series of fused vertebra that articulate with the lowest lumbar vertebra and both ilia as well as the coccyx.

> **ilia (singular, ilium):** Two irregularly shaped bones that articulate with the sacrum and house the hip socket where the femur

articulates. Other landmarks of the ilium are:

ASIS (anterior superior iliac spine): A landmark to which the tensor fascia lata attaches and below which the rectus femoris and sartorius muscles attach. This is the bony prominence on the upper front of the hip and an important landmark for assessing pelvic rotation.

symphysis pubis: A joint formed by the pubic bones of both ilia. The orientation of the ASIS and symphysis pubis determines whether the pelvis is anteriorly or posteriorly rotated (see related terms).

iliac crest: The top edge of the ilium. Feeling the iliac crests and comparing them side-to-side helps form a more complete picture of the pelvis's contribution to back pain or hip pain.

ischial tuberosity: The bony part of the ilium on which hamstring muscles originate. This is also commonly referred to as the "sit bone."

coccyx: Small, fused vertebrae attached to the sacrum.

posterior
Behind or in back of; the opposite of anterior. For instance, the heel of the foot is posterior to the toes.

pelvic tilt
The pelvis can rotate forward (anteriorly) or backward (posteriorly).

anterior pelvic tilt: The top of the pelvis is rotated forward. The effect of the anterior tilt increases spinal extension.

posterior pelvic tilt: The top of the pelvis is rotated back. The effect of the posterior tilt increases spinal flexion.

pronation
A rotational movement typically associated with the forearm and hand as well as the foot. Pronation of the foot occurs when the arch of the foot drops down closer to the floor. This is a natural occurrence during walking but in some people, the arch remains down; this is referred to as a pronated foot.

prone
Term given to the body position wherein a person is lying on their stomach.

quadriceps
Group of four thigh muscles that attach into the patella and extend the knee.

quadruped
Term given to the position wherein a person is on their hands and knees.

rectus abdominus—See abdominal muscles.

rectus femoris
One of the quadriceps muscles that originates below the ASIS of the ilium and inserts with the other quadriceps muscles into the patella. This muscle helps flex the hip joint as well as extend the knee.

retroversion (femoral)
A structural external twisting of the femur that points the knees outward when the femur is correctly aligned in the hip socket.

sacrum—See pelvis.

sartorius
A muscle originating at the ASIS of the pelvis and inserting below the knee joint onto the inner portion of the tibia. The sartorius flexes, externally rotates, and abducts the hip and flexes and internally rotates the knee joint.

sciatica
Irritation of the sciatic nerve causing pain in the buttocks or down the back of the leg, even into the foot.

sciatic nerve
A major nerve feeding the leg that originates in the lumbar vertebrae and travels down the back of the leg.

SI joint
The joint formed where the ilium meets the sacrum in the pelvis.

SI joint dysfunction
Pain located in the back of the pelvis around the SI joint.

supine
Term given to the body position wherein a person is lying on their back.

symphysis pubis—See pelvis.

tensor fascia lata (TFL)
Originates on the anterior portion of the iliac crest and ASIS and inserts into the ITB. It flexes, medially rotates, and abducts the leg and can cause pelvic rotation problems.

tibia
One of the lower leg bones that articulates with the femur to form the knee joint. The distal portion of the tibia forms the medial ankle bone.

transversus abdominus (TA)—See abdominal muscles.

About the Author

Rick Olderman MSPT, CPT

Following graduation in 1996 from the nationally ranked Krannert School of Physical Therapy at the University of Indianapolis, I practiced at a small sports and orthopedic clinic in Cortez, Colorado. Because the clinic had a small gym attached, I was able to progress patients to a higher functional level than if I were in a typical clinic. This unique model influenced me to consider personal training. I discovered that setting up therapeutic training programs for my patients helped them as much or more than any intervention I would perform manually.

I moved to Denver in 1999 and began working as a physical therapist and personal trainer at an exclusive health club, The Athletic Club at Denver Place. While there, I continued to experiment with blending rehabilitation and personal training and added Pilates to my skill set. Within just a few months, I became the top-producing employee at the club. I held that position for the next four years until I opened my own studio/clinic.

In addition to providing individual client services, I also lead corporate seminars for injury prevention and correction. My focus on teaching employees the fundamentals of injury mechanics and practical ways to correct them has made me an effective force in changing corporate thinking about injuries, injury prevention, ergonomics, and fitness programs. I believe education is the key. I find that if you teach someone how the body works and why they experience pain, most people will be more diligent in helping themselves. No one wants to be in pain.

I am an active member of the American Physical Therapy Association, and I continue to explore combined rehabilitation and fitness techniques through professional development and continuing education. I live and work in Denver, Colorado with my wife and two young children.

REFERENCES

Introduction opening quote:
Nechis, Barbara. 1993. *Watercolor from the Heart*. New York: Watson-Guptill Publications.

Section 1 opening quote:
Yogananda, Paramahansa. 1997. *Journey to Self-Realization*. Los Angeles, CA: Self-Realization Fellowship.

Section 2 opening quote:
Chopra, Deepak. 1993. *Creating Affluence: Wealth Consciousness in the Field of All Possibilities*. San Rafael, CA: New World Library.

Section 3 opening quote:
Campbell, Joseph. 1991. *The Joseph Campbell Companion: Reflections on the Art of Living*. Ed. Diane K. Osbon. New York: HarperCollins.

Kendall, Florence, Elizabeth McCreary, and Patricia Provance. 1993. *Muscles: Testing and Function, with Posture and Pain*. Fourth edition. Baltimore, MD: Williams & Wilkins.

Sahrmann, Shirley A. 2002. *Diagnosis and Treatment of Movement Impairment Syndromes*. St. Louis, MO: Mosby.

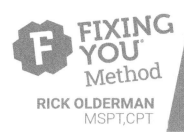
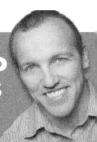
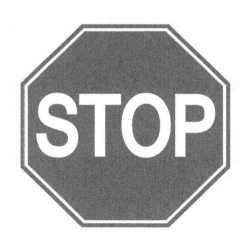

Made in the USA
Monee, IL
16 July 2022

99869947R00075